INTRODUCTION
To Long Term Care

Sometimes There Is No Choice

"Placing my mother in a nursing home was the hardest thing I've ever done. I cried all night."

Problem

Your loved one needs to be placed in a nursing home. **You are responsible**. No, you did not wish for the responsibility, but you must act. Your loved one is completely vulnerable and dependent on you. You must make the right choice about something which you have always heard about, but never wanted know about. You must find a good *nursing home*.

Resolution

You *can* do it, with the help of persons who have been this way before. There are professionals who can and want to help you. You may find the assistance of Elder law attorneys, Geriatric Case Managers, Nurses and Social Workers helpful at this time of one of the most difficult decisions in life. This booklet is but one example. It was put together by Jim Schuster, Certified Elder Law attorney, with the hope that it will give you information that will make this burden a little lighter. He has helped many and he hopes he will help you.

Copyright 2018
Jim Schuster, Certified Elder law Attorney
17436 College Parkway, Livonia MI 48152
(248) 356-3500 – www.JimSchuster.com

Copies of this publication are available
Please contact us at the address above

TABLE OF CONTENTS

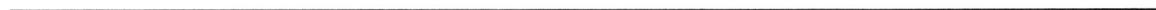

FORWARD

This book is addressed to two classes of nursing home residents: those in short term, post hospital care and the long term care nursing home resident. In the legal sense there is no distinction between the two. Both have the same rights. The difference lies in the cause for nursing home placement, the source of payment for the care and finally the expectations of the resident and family.

Most short term cases are caused by a medical condition that needs intensive treatment. This case may involve post hip surgery rehabilitative therapy, or treatment for an illness the patient should recover from such as pneumonia. The patient expects Medicare to cover the cost and to return to home.

Most long term care arises from conditions such as advanced dementia or major stroke where the patient's family cannot provide sufficient care at home. In these cases the family does not expect the patient to return to home. Medicare does not cover long term care.

There is a too common case where a short term stay turns into long term care. Sometimes the patient does not get better and in fact may get worse. Sometimes it should be expected: the patient may be sicker or weaker than thought. But, too often long term care results from preventable causes. One of the missions of this is to minimize these cases by empowering the Patient's Advocate to get the best of care.

We hope we have succeeded.

Terms – A note about terms.
"Patient advocate:" means any person who is assisting the patient with the management of healthcare. It might be one person or it might be a family team. However the person who is acting must have authority to speak for the patient. Note that under some usage the term is limited to mean the agent who speaks for the patient concerning end of life care, when the patient cannot speak for him or herself.

"Patient" and "Resident:" When we look to Medicare to pay the bill the person is a "patient." When a person is in a nursing home they have legal rights of a "resident." This is because the law reflects the old practice of using the nursing home as a home for the "resident." The law grants the patient or resident rights in the nursing home setting be it short term or long term care.

Gender: I often refer to the patient/resident in the female gender instead of switching between he and she. I use this device for ease and uniformity.

You Need Legal Authority
(Get it from the patient or the probate court)

If you have a family member in a hospital, you may be asked for papers to show your *legal authority to make decisions* for your loved one. It does not matter if you are husband, wife, parent or child - you need legal authority to make decisions for another. In addition to managing the delivery of healthcare you may be signing contracts, filing applications for assistance, filing tax returns or appealing a denial of benefits. You may have to withdraw funds from a brokerage account and sell property. You will need documents to prove your authority and if you have none, then either the patient must execute those or you will have to go to probate court. Proceeding without authority is risky. At a minimum you may find yourself paying expensive healthcare bills and at worst your family member's life may be at risk.

What do you need? You need either powers of attorney or be appointed the person's guardian by the probate court. Note that powers of attorney are narrowly read and only give the powers stated in the document. Nothing is implied. That means when it comes to making all decisions for another you need *complete* authority. If you don't have it you will need to get it from the probate court.

Can your patient give you legal authority if he or she has significant medical problems? If she can communicate with you the answer is likely "yes." Persons with only minimal capacity to make decisions, may give another authority to act for them.

Healthcare Power of Attorney
You should have a complete power of attorney to all make medical decisions. The power should be immediately effective. If it is not then it is "springing" and you have to satisfy the condition that causes it to spring into effect. A typical condition requires two doctor's letters declaring incapacity, before you can do anything.

A complete power of attorney authorizes medical providers to share confidential medical information covered by the privacy portions HIPAA law and the Michigan Medical Records Access Act. But you need more authority than to just receive information. You must have authority to make all decisions. That includes decisions about mental health care. Many times a patient/resident is referred to a psychiatrist for a behavior problem, such as depression, anxiety, side effects from medications and so on. You must have authority to consent and withdraw consent for such treatment. And, your authority must include end-of-life decision making.

You need the power to make all necessary medical decisions, including:

a. approve or refuse, consent or withdraw consent to, all types of medical care, treatment, and procedures;
b. be designated as the Health Insurance Portability and Accountability Act or "HIPAA" personal representative authorized to access medical records, disclose the contents to other medical providers, and execute medical releases;
c. authorize admission to or discharge from (even against medical advice) any hospital, nursing home, or care facility;
d. contract for any health care related service or facility, without incurring personal financial liability for such contracts;
e. hire and fire medical and other support personnel responsible for care;
f. execute documents including releases and refusal of treatment forms or do-not- resuscitate orders, that a facility may require to carry out patient instructions regarding medical treatment.

Designation of Patient Advocate

When it comes to end-of-life medical treatment decision making, Michigan has strict conditions for any power of attorney that would allow termination of life sustaining treatment. The law allows the creation of a document called a "designation of patient advocate." It is more than a "living will" that merely states a person's wishes for end of life care. It names the patient advocate(s), gives end-of-life decision making instructions, and gives the authority to make all necessary medical decisions.

The authority granted may only be exercised when two doctors have certified that the patient *unable to participate* in medical decision making.

The document must give instructions to the patient advocate as to when treatment may be terminated. The patient advocate may not make the decision on his/her own.

The document must state that the patient understands that termination of treatment *could allow death.*

The document must be signed by two witnesses who are not related to the patient, and do not work a healthcare facility where the patient is receiving treatment. A notarized signature will not suffice.

A Designation of Patient Advocate Is Limited to End-of-life Decision Making

When you are not dealing with end-of-life medical treatment you cannot rely on a Designation of Patient Advocate form from a hospital or nursing home. These generic forms address end-of-life medical treatment only. They are necessarily limited in scope and authority granted. These address who is the patient, who is the patient advocate, and what are the end-of-life instructions? What if the patient recovers from the "terminal" condition? These forms do not address ongoing care needs. They do not allow the patient advocate to participate in decision-making if the patient *can*. They do not address mental health treatment (e.g. depression, paranoia) or managing healthcare in general. Again, if you do not have the authority you need you will have to petition the probate court for the appointment of a guardian. Consult an elder law attorney to ensure that the document grants sufficient *immediate* authority for healthcare decisions. It should cover present needs as well as the end-of-life authority and instructions.

General Durable Power of Attorney

A general durable power of attorney is an authorization granted by a "principal" to an "agent," sometimes called an "attorney in fact." The agent can handle the all business of the principal, even if the principal is incapacitated. That is what "durable" means. The authority granted may include that to sign contracts, file applications or tax returns, appeal denial of benefits, and pay or contest bills. One Michigan probate judge observed that almost all guardian or conservator proceedings could be avoided by a durable power of attorney. A person need not be fully healthy to sign a power of attorney. He need have the mental capacity to be aware of his need for help, who he wants to help him, and what he wants that person to do.

The power of attorney only grants authority that is expressly given. A complete power of attorney must address all needs of the principal including retirement plans, insurance, credit cards, opening and closing accounts. An elder law focused power considers special powers such as the authority to make gifts, sell property to family members at discount, employ family members or draft a trust for an estate plan. While these powers may not be important to a healthy person, they can be invaluable for an elder to have her wishes carried out. An elder law attorney should be consulted for drafting a suitable and complete document.

Trustee Successorship

If the person you are helping has property in a trust, you may need to activate the successor trustee. You must review the trust for the procedure or consult an attorney to handle the review and necessary paperwork.

Guardianship

If you do not have power of attorney <u>and</u> your loved one does not have the minimal capacity to execute a power of attorney, you will need to "petition" the probate court for a hearing to be appointed *guardian* or *conservator*.

The *guardian* makes the personal decisions for the such as what medical treatment will be needed, who will administer the treatment, and where the ward will reside. The *conservator* makes the financial decisions and handles the money. Both guardian and conservator report to the probate court. One person may handle both roles. The appointment of a full guardian or conservator removes the legal right of the patient to make decisions.

The *petition* is a form available at the county probate court. You may complete it yourself, or you may have a social worker who can complete it. The petition must be correctly completed and filed at the probate court. Of course, you may hire an attorney who will complete and file the petition and represent you in court at the hearing. You can ask the court to have the patient repay you.

The filing fee is $150 for guardian or conservator. The court will schedule a hearing within four to eight weeks, unless there is an emergency in which case the court can appoint a temporary guardian. An emergency means that the person's health or finances are at risk for immediate harm. An example might be emergency surgery is needed. There is a $20 additional fee for emergency petitions.

The court will appoint a *guardian ad litem*. This is an attorney who will make an investigation and file a report with the court. This attorney will speak to the petitioner and the alleged incapacitated person, and make any other needed inquiry to report whether the petition should be approved and whether the proposed ward objects or agrees. The fee for the guardian ad litem may range from $350 to $600 in uncontested matters and may go higher.

On the hearing date the judge will decide whether a guardian/conservator should be appointed and, if so, who that person should be. The "alleged legally incapacitated person" may agree or object. If there is any contest on the need for a guardian/conservator, the judge will hold a hearing. When the court appoints a guardian or conservator it issues *letters of authority*. These spell out the authority given. The guardian and conservator are subject to the supervision of the probate court and must file annual reports. The conservator files an inventory and annual accounting. The guardian files a report of the person's condition.

Guardianship Or?

Given that full guardianship *removes the rights of an individual to make decisions,* and the costs of obtaining guardianship – the filing fee, the guardian ad litem fee, time off work and costs of a private attorney – many people ask, "What are my alternatives?" This is a legitimate question, since the law requires the probate court to inform petitioners for appointment of a guardian of the alternatives to public-court supervision. The court carries out its mandate by Probate Court Form 666, see: courts.mi.gov/Administration/SCAO/Forms/courtforms/guardian-conservator/pc 666.pdf

What are the alternatives? As stated in Michigan Probate Court Form 666 they are:

1. **Health Care Power of Attorney.** There are two types: a *patient advocate designation* and a *durable power of attorney for health care.*

2. **Do-Not-Resuscitate Order.** A do-not-resuscitate order is a document directing that the patient named in the order not be resuscitated if the patient's spontaneous respiration and circulation stop in a setting outside a medical facility.

3. **Durable Power of Attorney.** A power of attorney is a document signed by a competent person giving another person the power to manage some or all of his or her affairs.

4. **Trust.** A trust may be a substitute for a conservator and a will. The trust expresses the desires of the maker (called a *settlor*) about the management of his or her assets during his or her lifetime and when physically or mentally unable to manage the assets.

The court recognizes that the powers of attorney are affordable alternatives to court proceedings. But what if a person is no longer competent? PC 666 recognizes the following alternatives to full guardianship even if the individual is mentally incapable of making decisions.

1. **Limited Guardian.** A guardian who makes only those decisions for the individual that the court allows.

2. **Conservator.** A conservator is a person appointed by probate court and given power and responsibility for the estate (financial assets and property) of an adult (called a *protected individual*).

3. **Protective Order.** When only a single transaction affecting the property of a disabled person is required, the probate court may enter a protective order for this one time matter without appointing a conservator or a guardian.

4. **Representative Payee.** A representative payee is appointed by the Social Security Administration to handle benefits. There is no court involvement. The representative payee's authority is limited to the benefits.

5. **Special Services for the Aging.** Many communities have voluntary services available upon request to help the aging with their financial affairs.

Seniors are glad to retain their independence and use one of these alternatives.

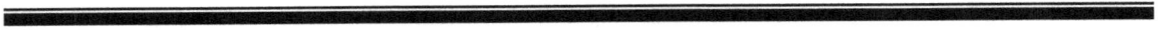

How to Get Good Care

1. First: you must have recognizable authority to act for the person. Being a spouse, child or sibling is not enough. You need a medical/healthcare power of attorney signed by the patient. Broadly speaking in Michigan there are two types: The "designation of patient advocate," commonly known as a living will, and the general healthcare power of attorney.

The "designation of patient advocate" concerns end of life medical treatment. The authority is effective only when two doctors certify that the patient cannot participate in informed medical decision making.

The general healthcare power of attorney can and should be an immediately effective, durable power of attorney. Durable means it is still effective even though the patient may be incapacitated. It does not need doctor's certification and it grants authority to make any and all medical decisions for the patient. You need the second one to be empowered to act for the patient.

2. The advocate must "manage" the patient's care. That means being fully advised of the current treatment plan and making sure it is fully carried out. It means asking questions. It means being vigilant for problems not being treated such as a developing bedsore or reaction to a new medication. It means talking to staff and the doctor about treatment issues. It means getting your patient to emergency if serious medical problems are not immediately addressed.

Good care requires active management of the delivery of healthcare. Remember: You are the boss. You are employing them to provide care to your patient.

3. Whether you are acting for the patient in home, in hospital or in a nursing home you need to be informed. In any setting you must know the patient's rights and actively exercise them. In home, hospital or nursing home that means knowing the patient's rights and benefits under Medicare. See the Medicare section of this book.

In the nursing home the patient a long list of rights granted by the Nursing Home Reform Act. These include the right to make medical treatment decisions; the right: to be fully informed in advance of any changes in care or treatment; the right to accept or refuse medical treatment; the right to choose your own doctor. You can read more below "Nursing Home Residents' Rights."

4. When it comes to nursing home care you must choose the best facility you can. Medicare rates nursing homes on a number of factors that measure quality of care.

You can find the nursing home ratings on the Medicare website, Medicare.gov. Look for section that covers "Find doctors, providers, hospitals, plans & suppliers" and choose "find a nursing home." There you will be able to see a list of nursing homes in your area and review the quality scores. Medicare rates homes by a star system. 5 Star homes are the best. 1 Star is the worst. 5 Star homes can be hard to find, 1 Star homes must be avoided.

Since most nursing homes fall in the average 3 Star range, the most important factor is daily visitation. You would rather have a 2 Star home where you could visit daily, and quickly in case of emergency, rather than a 4 Star home you could only visit on the weekends.

5. Find out who is the representative of the Long Term Care Ombudsman assigned to your nursing home. You may find that it is difficult to make any changes in the institutional care your patient is getting. What if the nursing home staff do not listen? Is it "your word against theirs?" No.

Under the Nursing Home Reform Law of 1987 the people in nursing homes have guaranteed rights. It surprises many but a resident is supposed to be able to choose his or her activities (including bedtime) and have veto power over a treatment plan. This runs counter to the common experience of institutional care that most experience. Everybody gets up at the same time. In the evening its lights out at the same time. And so on.

How does the advocate have any leverage against the institutional "system?" Know who is the Long Term Care Ombudsman representative that covers your nursing home. Their role is to improve the quality of care and quality of life experienced by residents who reside in licensed long term care facilities. Part of that includes informing nursing homes when they out of compliance with the law and regulations concerning resident care and rights.

For example we had a situation where a shiny new nursing home proposed discharge a resident to another nursing home after he completed his post-hospital skilled care covered by Medicare. We informed the advocate that the resident had a right to stay there and apply for Medicaid. The nursing home thought they could choose who they would offer the Medicaid beds to. We had the advocate contact the Long Term Care Ombudsman's office and the nursing home was set straight. The resident stayed.

So know who the Long Term Care Ombudsman representative is for your nursing home. Their number is 1–866-485-9393.

Post Hospital Care

A short term stay in a nursing home is most often preceded by hospital treatment. But, long term care often begins in the hospital as well. There are a number of reasons. An elder may suffer a fall requiring surgery, then recuperation does not go well enough for a return to home. It may be a major stroke requiring care beyond that can be provided at home. Post surgical complications may develop into long term care. Often Alzheimer's Dementia becomes much worse after a hospital stay. Sometimes the hospital stay makes a caregiver, most often a spouse, step back and realize he cannot do it anymore.

There are practical reasons for the hospital stay to be the beginning of long term care. First it is a much easier transition for the elder/patient and much easier for the family to go from home to hospital. The second is that the hospital discharge planners have the duty to find an open bed at a nursing home. That makes it much easier on the family who would otherwise have to go driving around to nursing homes with the medical and financial information for the nursing home to review. Often families are told there is a year waiting list only to find that a call from "Big Hospital" gets immediate placement and the waiting list disappears.

A hospital is under great pressure to discharge because once the treatment is done, Medicare stops paying. The discharge planner may just say to the nursing home "Take this one as a favor to us. We'll make it up later." The downside of the hospital making placement is that it may make placement at a facility it regularly does business with. The placement may be at a nursing home that does not have open long term care beds, yet the patient needs long term care. Finally the nursing home may not be the patient and family's first choice. You always have the right to arrange a better placement

The Patient Advocate and the Rights of the Medicare Patient
Even if the resident did not enter a nursing home from the hospital, the patient advocate must be knowledgeable about Medicare processes. A long term nursing home resident may have trips to the hospital. When the resident enters the nursing home on a post-hospital skilled care stay, the quality and completeness of treatment may dictate how well the patient does. Sometimes the patient returns home only through the vigorous advocacy of the patient advocate. The patient advocate is essential to the patient receiving quality care.

Written Notice of Patient's Rights
Medicare participating hospitals must deliver written notice, the *Important Message from Medicare*, of a patient's rights as a hospital patient including discharge appeal rights, at or near admission. The notice must contain the following essential pieces

of information:

- The name(s) of the patient's physician(s) and the patient's ID number.
- A statement of the right to file an appeal or raise questions with the Medicare Quality Improvement Organization (QIO) about quality of care, including hospital discharge.
- The name and telephone number of the QIO that serves the area in which the hospital in question is located.
- A space for the beneficiary or representative to sign and date the document.
- The steps necessary to appeal a hospital discharge decision or to file a complaint about the quality of care.

Premature hospital discharge

In the context of this publication a premature discharge may occur when the patient still needs hospital care or when the proposed discharge plan is inappropriate. If a person is too ill or weak to return to home where there is not enough support, then discharge to home care is inappropriate. The at-home spouse may not be able to care for the hospital spouse because of her own medical problems. Sending the patient home in that case leads to emergency return to the hospital, often with even worse problems such as a broken hip from a fall.

The Medicare patient has the right to appeal premature termination of hospital benefits. The entire complex and lengthy appeal process may proceed through the levels of "review", reconsideration, Administrative Law Judge hearing, Appeal Council review and finally federal district court. The patient advocate may be most effective at the time of notice of discharge, which is the review stage. We will focus on this latter point.

Follow Procedure in the "Important Message from Medicare" Notice

The advocate must follow the procedures in the *Important Message from Medicare* Notice. This form is given to the hospital patient on admission. There are <u>very strict and short time lines</u>. The advocate must request a review either orally or in writing no later than the day of discharge. A "timely" request is no later than midnight of the <u>day of discharge and before leaving the hospital</u>. The request is made with **KEPRO**, the Quality Improvement Organization (QIO) for Michigan. Once this is done the patient may remain in the hospital without charge at least until noon of the day after the QIO review decision. Contact **KEPRO** at (855) 408-8557.

Immediately Contact the Patient's Physician

Without missing the "same day" deadline, above, the advocate must also *immediately* contact the physician in charge of the patient. This doctor is the "attending physician" assigned by the hospital. If the doctor does not agree with the discharge plan, the doctor then must advise the hospital Utilization Review Committee. Often the discharge is stopped at this point. If the hospital proposes to continue with the discharge, it must then present its decision and the patient's record to KEPRO for review

It is vital to present to the patient's doctor the reasons why the termination of hospital coverage is wrong. Where the discharge is ill advised the decision to discharge may well be more related to the Medicare payment system than the needs of the patient. Medicare pays for services according to treatment group and that means that some patients need more care and others need less. That creates an incentive to provide less care. However the Medicare benefit covers all medical care that is reasonable and necessary for hospital treatment of the patient. The advocate must advocate for the individual needs of the patient.

Prepare Your Case for Review
Many QIO reviews fail the patient because of inadequate preparation. The Centers for Medicare Advocacy have a self help packet of information you *need to know*. http://www.medicareadvocacy.org/self-help-packet-for-expedited-skilled-nursin g-facility-appeals-including-improvement-standard-denials/

Payment for Hospital Expenses During Review
Patients are *not* financially liable for hospital costs incurred during the KEPRO review; they are responsible only for coinsurance and deductibles. If the KEPRO decision is in agreement with the hospital (unfavorable to the patient), then the patient becomes liable for the medical expenses incurred beginning at noon on the *day after* notification of the decision is given.

Inappropriate Discharge
What if the patient agrees with discharge but disagrees with the discharge plan? For example, what if, as mentioned above, the plan is to discharge to home where the spouse is unable to meet the recuperative needs of the patient? Medicare *requires* a discharge plan that is appropriate to the patient. Or, suppose a patient needs skilled nursing care but a bed is not available locally. Medicare coverage can continue until the appropriate discharge may be made. That means the hospital may not discharge a patient to a nursing home so many miles away that family cannot visit. Again, such a decision could be reason for a KEPRO Review of the discharge plan.

Discharge Planning
(A critical step too often poorly executed)

Discharge Planning Evaluation[1]
Medicare requires an evaluation of the needs of the patient before making a discharge plan. The patient's physician may order the planning. The plan must assess the feasibility of the patient returning to his home. It must reassess the plan if it is inappropriate. It must identify the skilled nursing facilities available to the patient for skilled care. The regulation is found at 42 CFR 482.43.

The Right of the Hospital Patient to Discharge Planning
Medicare requires that the hospital patient be discharged according to an appropriate care plan. The hospital must identify at an early stage of hospitalization all patients who are likely to suffer adverse health consequences upon discharge if there is not adequate discharge plan. A plan may also be requested. The components of the process are:
(1) The hospital must provide a discharge planning evaluation upon the patient's request, the request of a person acting on the patient's behalf, or the request of the physician.
(2) A registered nurse, social worker, or other appropriately qualified personnel must develop, or supervise the development of, the evaluation.
(3) The discharge planning evaluation must include an evaluation of the likelihood of a patient needing post- hospital services and of the availability of the services.
(4) The discharge planning evaluation must include an evaluation of the likelihood of a patient's capacity for self-care or of the possibility of the patient being cared for in the environment from which he or she entered the hospital.
(5) The hospital personnel must complete the evaluation on a timely basis so that appropriate arrangements for post-hospital care are made before discharge, and to avoid unnecessary delays in discharge.
(6) The hospital must include the discharge planning evaluation in the patient's medical record for use in establishing an appropriate discharge plan and must discuss the results of the evaluation with the patient or individual acting on his or her behalf.

This includes consideration of more than medical treatment. For the patient who requires skilled nursing care, the discharge must be to a nursing facility within a "reasonable" area. A nursing home placement that would cut the patient off from

---

[1]Note: I have provided references to law and regulation for some of the points below. I do this for two reasons: 1) these statements are not "just my opinion" and 2) you can "look it up" and prove it if you meet resistance. CFR means Code of Federal Regulations. USC stands for United States Code, the compilation of the laws of the US government.

family and community support is inappropriate and could be medically harmful. What if the hospital cannot find an appropriate placement?

Medicare law provides for continued hospital care if the patient requires skilled nursing care and no appropriate bed is available. 42 U.S.C.1395x(v)(1)(G)(i), 42 CFR412.42(c)(1), 412.80(a)(1), 424.13(b). The primary burden of locating a bed is placed on the hospital. 42 USC 1395x(ee), 42 CFR 412.12(b). Because of the financial pressure to discharge patients, this requirement is often ignored by hospital staff.

Given the difficulties some patients face in securing a skilled nursing facility bed following hospitalization, this is an area where appeals are often appropriate. Financial difficulties, including problems relating to securing eligibility for Medicaid are not valid reasons for denying Medicare coverage. The sole issue is whether the patient was offered placement in an appropriate Medicare-certified Skilled nursing facility. Timely appeals of notice of discharge are made to the **(KEPRO) (855) 408-8557** .

The primary burden of locating a skilled nursing facility bed is placed on the treating physician, 42 CFR 412.12(b), and on the hospital discharge planner, 42 U.S.C. 1395x(ee). Patients and their families need only cooperate with the efforts of the hospital discharge planning staff. However the advocate will want to personally inspect any facility to be assured that it *will* provide the requisite level of care and is reasonably close to the patient's home or family so that daily visits are possible.

Whether a person is in a hospital or a nursing home, the law requires "discharge planning." It is a plan of care and treatment made specially for the patient. This involves more than mere "transfer." A facility may not say words to the effect "He will be in the lobby at noon." In practice, discharge planning is a mix of commonsense actions and procedures required by law.

When the planning is properly completed, the patient/resident will have been involved in decisions about what will take place after leaving the facility. The patient may request assistance in arranging necessary services prior to discharge. For example, if the person is going home, the plan may include obtaining transportation to the scheduled follow-up appointment with the doctor.

The patient or advocate should have answers to important questions prior to leaving the facility. The plan must address:
  where the patient is going after the facility and what will happen after arrival;
  the medication regimen including how to obtain and administer;
  the name and phone number of a person to contact should problem arise during transfer;
  the potential side effects of medication and who to call if they occur;

what symptoms to watch out for and who to call should they arise;

how to keep the health problems from becoming worse;

if the patient is going home, whether there is someone to support the patient at home who knows what will be needed.

For any follow-up or referral appointment, the patient must know the time, date, location and who the appointment is with.

The above is adapted from the discharge preparation checklist by Dr. Eric Coleman, UCHSC, HCPR.

Legal Issues

Discharge planning is a formal process required by law. Resident records should contain a final resident discharge summary which addresses the resident's post-discharge needs *(42 CFR §483.20(l))*. Facilities must identify patients who are likely to suffer adverse health consequences in the absence of discharge planning services. They must develop plan of care with the participation of the resident and family. The plan must be designed to assist the resident to adjust to his or her living environment. This applies to discharges to home, to a nursing facility, or to another type of residential facility such as assisted living. *(42 CFR §483.20(l))*.

A proposed discharge may not be appropriate. It may be too soon, the patient is not healthy enough, or necessary post-hospital services have not been arranged. A discharge of a long term care patient to a nursing home without open Medicaid beds is inappropriate. If the problem cannot be resolved prior to the discharge date, the advocate may ask for review. That is done through the local Quality Improvement Organization (QIO). The patient's hospital discharge <u>notice</u> should provide the name, address, and phone number of the QIO serving the hospital, along with instructions on how to ask for review *(42 CFR §§412.42-412.48)*. **KEPRO** is the QIO in Southeast Michigan. Contact them by (855) 408-8557 or by <u>www.KEPRO.com.</u>

Time to Change Your Medicare Provider?

What if the patient's Medicare Advantage provider does not cover all nursing homes? You may not be able to secure Medicare paid treatment in a local nursing home. A little known fix is that a patient in a hospital or nursing home can change to traditional Medicare at any time and go back to the HMO after the treatment is completed. Just enroll in traditional Medicare before the end of the month, early enough to change the official record, and your patient will have a choice of any nursing home to provide her Medicare benefit. After the treatment is over simply re-enroll in your chosen Medicare Advantage plan.

The Medicare Benefit

One of the most important subjects the patient advocate must know about is the post-hospital Medicare "skilled care" benefit in a skilled nursing facility. This is a *100 day maximum* benefit. All skilled nursing facilities are nursing homes. It does not matter whether the facility refers to itself as a "rehabilitation center" or a "short term care facility." If it is not licensed as a *nursing home* then Medicare will not pay.

A Patient Advocate must know what "skilled care" is. If the nursing home care is not "skilled" then it is considered "custodial" or "personal" care and Medicare will not pay. One may think that all care in a nursing home is skilled care since a nursing home is a licensed medical facility with trained, certified, medical personnel. That may be true but when it comes to the Medicare benefit if the care is not "skilled" such as performed by a nurse or a therapist, then Medicare will not pay for the nursing home. But, even if the patient receives skilled care, it is possible for Medicare to refuse payment.

The "Observation Status" problem: Medicare will not pay for post-hospital skilled care:

Medicare will not pay for post-hospital skilled nursing care in a nursing home unless there was a hospital "admission." That is not the same as a hospital "stay." There are three conditions that must be met by the hospital before Medicare will pay. First, the patient must have been "admitted"; second, the patient must have stayed three days; third, the patient must be discharged with an order for skilled care. We will cover the first two and then discharge orders later.

Medicare A and Medicare B

The Observation Status issue is whether Medicare A will pay for the hospital stay and post hospital skilled care in a nursing home. Thus, this discussion is about Medicare coverage, not medical terminology. If medical treatment is not covered under Medicare A then only some of it will be covered under Medicare B. We might understand the difference as Medicare A pays for "inpatient" hospital care and Medicare B will only pay for "out patient" services. Only Medicare A pays for post hospital skilled nursing care. To trigger a claim under Medicare A the patient must be "admitted" to the hospital.

"Admission to Hospital"

This term has caused great confusion, denials of coverage, cases in court and Congressional hearings and action. For the lay person the term "admission" has changed in definition. It used to be that if you got a bed in a hospital you were "admitted." Now, for purposes of the Medicare benefit you may not have been admitted, you received "out patient" services. These are not covered under *Medicare*

A. Only "in patient" services are covered.

"Observation Status"

Most people know that treatment in the "emergency room" is not admission to the hospital. In Medicare terminology the person is an "outpatient" and Medicare will pay emergency room services under Medicare B. Where it gets confusing is the situation where the patient leaves the emergency room to a bed in another part of the hospital. Are they "admitted"? CMS, the Medicare agency, gives this example:

> You visit the ED and are sent to the intensive care unit
> (ICU) for close monitoring. Your doctor expects you to be
> sent home the next morning unless your condition worsens.
> Your condition resolves and you're sent home the next day.

In this case Medicare deems you an outpatient. You are not an inpatient and you have not been admitted to the hospital. Your stay in ICU was for "observation." While the answer makes sense, what if you stay in the hospital for three more days while the doctors take tests and wait for lab results? Then what if the doctor decides that you need rehab therapy and discharges you to a skilled care facility for rehab? Medicare will not pay for the nursing home because you did not receive care covered under Medicare A. Your treatment will be covered under Medicare B, which is not a hospital benefit. This sort of thing has happened.

Confusion arises when the patient leaves the hospital emergency department and "gets a bed upstairs" for purposes of "observation." This is not "admission" to the hospital. The hospital care for "observation" may not be billed under Medicare A, but rather Medicare B.

Medicare B does not pay for post-hospital skilled care in a nursing home. The "gotcha" is that Medicare A will not pay for post-hospital nursing home care unless the patient's hospital stay was covered under Medicare A, e.g. admitted as an "inpatient." That does mean that a patient could spend five days in the hospital and still not meet the Medicare 3 day hospital stay requirement of Medicare A.

CMS began to hear many citizen complaints and lawsuits over cases where patients were in the hospital as long as *eight days* and on discharge got an order for skilled care in a nursing home. After weeks in the nursing home they were shocked to hear that Medicare would not pay and that they owed the nursing home thousands of dollars. The reason? Medicare said they were never admitted as an inpatient. They were in for observation and that is an outpatient service.

The best practice to ask is whether your patient is classified as an inpatient or outpatient. If an outpatient and you anticipate long term care, ask the doctor why he or she did not write an order for admission as an inpatient and ask the doctor to order admission as inpatient.

"Three Days"
Medicare counts days as changing at mid-night so the requirement may be understood as *three midnights*. For example two people arrive in emergency 15 minutes apart. The first, after the usual hours and hours of waiting, is admitted at 11:50 p.m. The day of arrival at emergency is the first "day." The second is processed and admitted at 12:05 a.m. The time spent in Emergency does not count.

The Medicare post-hospital skilled nursing benefit secured
Once the patient meets the Medicare A requirements, e.g. 1) admission to the hospital, 2) three day stay in the hospital, 3) discharge with an order for skilled care, then the Medicare benefit is secured.

Medicare will pay the full cost of the nursing home stay for the first 20 days and will continue to pay the cost of the nursing home stay for the next 80 days, but with a deductible $167.50 per day (2018). Medicare supplemental insurance will pay the deductible. In order to qualify for the maximum 100 day benefit the patient must continue to need *skilled* care.

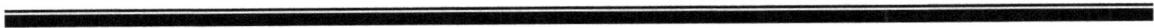

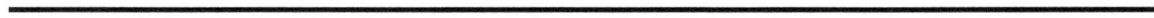

Get the Most out of Your Medicare Benefit

What is *skilled care*? Skilled care is service so inherently complex that it can be safely and effectively performed only by, or under the supervision of, professional or technical personnel. The skilled care may be for therapy, such as in the case of a broken hip. It may be medical as overcoming a severe infection. But, basic medical care, even in a nursing home, is not skilled care.

For example, a plaster cast on a leg does not usually require skilled care. However, if the patient has a pre-existing acute skin condition or needs traction, skilled personnel may be needed to adjust traction or watch for complications. In situations of this type, the complications, and the skilled services they require, must be documented by physicians' orders and nursing or therapy notes.

When it comes to choosing a nursing home the Medicare skilled benefit is an important unspoken consideration. For example, where a patient is in the nursing home for post-hospital rehabilitation the compensation for the nursing home can vary from $300 to over $700 per day. That makes the patient very attractive to any nursing home.

The higher payments are connected to intensive rehabilitation services. For example 720 minutes or more (total) of therapy per week in at least two disciplines is "Ultra High Intensity." 500 minutes or more (total) of therapy per week in at least one discipline for at least 5 days is "Very High Intensity." 325 minutes or more of therapy in at least one discipline for at least 5 days is High Intensity.

The patient advocate may take away two points: first, the more intense the work the better chance of improvement; second, the more the facility may receive the more attractive the person is as a resident. This last point is an often unspoken bargaining chip you have to get your person into the nursing home of your choice. That choice might be exercised at the initial placement or could be used for transfer to another nursing home.

The quality of patient advocacy can determine the quality of the outcome. The first, official, stage for patient advocacy comes in the care plan setting.

Care Plan for Post Hospital Skilled Care and Long Term Care

Medicare requires a care plan in a skilled nursing facility. But, care planning applies to both short-term, post-hospital and long term care. All nursing home residents must have a care plan. The Nursing Home Reform Law of 1987 was passed to improve the care of nursing home residents. The law requires that nursing home care result in improvement, if it is possible. Where improvement is not possible, the care must maintain abilities or slow the loss of function. It requires individualized care planning to meet these requirements. That process is made of the following components.

Care planning is most formal and "visible" during the Medicare skilled care benefit period. The patient advocate needs to be familiar with it, especially when there are patient issues that need attention.

The Care Planning Process
The delivery of the Medicare post-hospital skilled benefit is determined by the care plan assessment and report. For example, the team assesses and reports the extent of and the minutes per week of therapy received. The second component is accurately identifying the amount of assistance the patient needs with ADLs (Activities of Daily Living).

Federal Regulation – The Comprehensive Assessment.
The care planning process involves the initial assessment and periodic comprehensive re-assessments, of the functional capacity and needs of each resident. It is to take place within 14 days of admission. If the resident's physical or mental condition significantly changes, a re-assessment is required. The assessment must be accurate, comprehensive and standardized. 42 Code of Federal Regulation (CFR) 483.20.

Federal Regulation – The Comprehensive Care Plan.
42 CFR 483.20 (k) requires the care planning process to result in a comprehensive care plan for each resident. The plan must include measurable objectives and timetables to meet a resident's medical, nursing, mental and psycho-social needs as identified in the comprehensive assessment. The care plan must address
    (i) The services that are to be furnished to attain or maintain the resident's highest practicable physical, mental, and psycho-social well-being; and
    (ii) Any services that would otherwise be required under but are not provided due to the resident's exercise of rights including the right to refuse treatment.
    (2) A comprehensive care plan must be--
    (i) Developed within 7 days after completion of the comprehensive assessment;
    (ii) Prepared by an interdisciplinary team, that includes the attending physician, a registered nurse with responsibility for the resident, and other appropriate staff in disciplines as determined by the resident's needs, and, to the extent practicable, the participation of the resident, the resident's family or the resident's legal representative; and
    (iii) Periodically reviewed and revised by a team of qualified persons after each assessment.
42 CFR 483.20 (k)(2).

Long Term Care

The second role of the assessment is to define the care plan and provide a base for determining the patient's progress toward or decline from the care plan standard. The input of the patient advocate is critical. The team does not know how the patient was before: was he active or did he sit in the recliner all day? Was he happy or always cranky? They need your input.

How Care Planning Works in Practice

Every resident must have a treatment plan tailored to their individual needs. This includes the personal, as well as medical dimension. A person with profound hearing loss will not respond if her hearing aids are lost. She may be considered demented and unable to communicate. Staff must be sure she has her hearing aids and must be sure they have her attention when they speak to her. Most people with hearing loss must first see a person's face before they can hear them. A person Alzheimer's dementia may worsen after placement. Her confusion may increase to the point she stops responding or becomes agitated and aggressive. The care plan should include steps to improve the resident's adaptation and staff knowledge of her individual needs.

The care plan must not only the resident's present medical needs but must meet all needs. A person can lose the ability to walk if they remain in bed or a wheelchair 24 hours a day. A person can become incontinent if they are give a "diaper" and never taken to the bathroom when needed. A diabetic can suffer severe consequences if her medication regimen is not followed. These are just examples of the conditions that must be addressed in a resident's care plan.

A care plan must be able to change as needed. A patient who loses bladder control after entry into the nursing home has experienced a significant change in status. The staff must develop a new care plan that addresses this new need. For long term care residents the care plan must be reassessed, not just reviewed, annually.

The Assessment Team. The care plan is developed by a team from the nursing home, which may include a doctor, nurse, social worker, dietitian and physical, occupational or recreational therapist. They not only use medical information but must consider input from both the resident and the family about the resident's medical and emotional needs.

The Patient Advocate's Role. Your role is to be in charge of the care. You must first make your family member a person to the team, not just a "chart." You want to be sure they know his/her personality, values and abilities. You need to have a goal in mind for the facility. What should they accomplish? Is it return to home? Is it adaptation to long term care? They need your input. The advocate should be sure to inform the team of any allergies or adverse reactions to medications the resident may have. The scope of the assessment includes the resident's psychological, spiritual and social needs. The advocate should contribute information about the patient's preferences and routines. For example, is the resident usually talkative and social or more reclusive?

Your Input to the Assessment Team. During the assessment process, the patient advocate provides personal information beyond the hospital discharge order. For example, you may have noticed signs of depression along with symptoms of Alzheimer's. The assessment team may not notice these signs, so your input will be invaluable. Before the meeting, make a list of the resident's:

Medical needs; Psychological needs; Spiritual needs; Social needs; Preferences and usual routines; Dietary preferences; Items that could be lost, such as eyeglasses, hearing aides, or false teeth; anything else you deem important (It's easy to forget something in the pressure of a meeting!).

The team must be informed of factors that may affect the resident's behavior and what has worked before to address problems. A daughter might inform "Mother cannot hear without her hearing aid. She gets embarrassed about her inability to hear, so if she does not hear and understand something she will act as if she heard nothing at all." Without that information a staff person may think there is no point trying to talk with her since she does not understand.

Rule to remember: Only you know the patient. The care plan team does not. You know what she was capable of before entry into the hospital or nursing home. You should make sure the staff sets realistic goals - they should neither be too high nor too low. If too high the patient may be quickly seen as not suitable for rehabilitation. If too low, therapy will be terminated before the patient makes all the progress he or she could. For example your patient may have a broken hip. As patient advocate you might inform the team "Dad was walking before he fell and broke his hip. We expect him to walk out of the nursing home." Take special notice that a care plan may call for *rehabilitation* and *return to home*. It need not plan for a long term stay. Remember a return to home means the patient's home. If it has steps then the therapy must include the ability to get up the steps.

The assessment team uses the information they gather to develop an individualized formal care plan. The care plan defines specific needs of the resident and how the staff will meet them. The assessment team meets during the first month of a new resident's placement. The patient advocate *must* attend since the resident likely cannot or if s/he attends s/he may be too passive. Do not be passive, be active. Remember, you have hired them to help you.

The Care Plan Team. When you go to the care plan meeting keep in mind the goal you believe should be met by the therapy. Is it return to home or assisted living?

Is it adaptation to long term care? Whatever the desired result, bring along a copy of the list of needs you gave the assessment team earlier. Together, you can discuss your loved one's needs and the care plan the team has developed. And, if some need has been overlooked, you can ensure that the assessment team addresses it during this meeting.

The care plan becomes part of the nursing home contract. It should detail the resident's medical, emotional and social needs and spell out what will be done to improve or maintain the resident's health. The goals should not be too low - that can make the difference between a using a wheelchair and walking. If the goal is to return to home, then the resident *must be rehabilitated* enough to live at home with the support that is there.

Use the Care Plan. The patient advocate must monitor the patient's care to be sure the nursing home is following the plan. The advocate will attend all care planning meetings and give input on where the plan is succeeding and where it is not. The advocate can call for a specially convened conference because of a change in health. The affirmative use of the care planning process is the best way to ensure that the patient gets personal and appropriate care in the nursing home and achieves the highest level of functioning.

No "Improvement Standard" for Medicare Covered Therapy

It used to be common to hear that a patient's Medicare covered therapy was being discontinued because the patient had "plateaued" or "was not improving." This should no longer be the case since the settlement in *Jimmo v. Sebelius*, a nationwide class action case, in 2014. The question is whether the skilled services of a health care professional are medically necessary, not whether the beneficiary will "Improve." Persons with chronic conditions such as Alzheimer's should not be denied coverage for critical services because their underlying conditions will not improve. CMS, the federal agency responsible for Medicare, has issued conforming guidance to Medicare providers.

The restoration potential of a patient is not the deciding factor in determining whether skilled services are needed. Even if full recovery or medical improvement is not possible, a patient may need skilled services to prevent further deterioration or preserve current capabilities. 42 CFR 409.32(c).

While there is no "improvement standard" Medicare does require proof that skilled care is necessary. Medicare stipulates that coverage will "not be available in a situation where the beneficiary's maintenance care needs can be addressed safely and effectively through the use of nonskilled personnel." This means that the clinical record must support the need and the provider must bill Medicare appropriately as either rehabilitative or maintenance therapy. As Medicare says in its "Jimmo v. Sebelius Settlement Agreement Program Manual Clarifications Fact Sheet"

"In the case of *rehabilitative therapy*, the patient's condition has the potential to improve or is improving in response to therapy; maximum improvement is yet to be attained; and, there is an expectation that the anticipated improvement is attainable in a reasonable and generally predictable period of time. "

"In the case of *maintenance therapy*, the skills of a therapist are necessary to maintain, prevent, or slow further deterioration of the patient's functional status, and the services cannot be safely and effectively carried out by the beneficiary personally, or with the assistance of non-therapists, including unskilled caregivers."

Appeal Premature Termination of Medicare Coverage

What if you and the patient believe she needs skilled care and coverage is denied *before completion of 100 days*? In general we always recommend review by the Medicare QIO. It is quick, free and often easier to work out the problem at the earliest level. Appeal is a more serious undertaking. It requires the service be first provided and then a Medicare denial of payment-coverage for an expense already incurred. Then after you incurred the bill for services you can appeal. An appeal is an expensive undertaking that should only be done with complete preparation.

A Quick Screen for Review/Appeal of Termination of Medicare Coverage

(Reprinted by permission of the Center For Medicare Advocacy, Inc. Copyright)

1. The physician must certify that the patient needs skilled care.
2. The patient must require "skilled nursing or skilled rehabilitation services, or both, on a daily basis."

–Points to Consider on Appeal

1. The restoration potential of a patient is not the deciding factor.
2. The management of a plan of only various "custodial" personal care services is skilled when, in light of the patient's condition, the aggregate of those services requires the involvement of skilled personnel.
3. The requirement of "daily" skilled service is met if skilled *rehabilitation* services are provided five days a week.
4. Examples of skilled services:
   a. overall management and evaluation of the care plan;
   b. observation and assessment of the patient's changing condition;
   c. Levin tube and gastrostomy feedings;
   d. ongoing assessment of rehabilitation needs and potential;
   e. therapeutic exercises or activities;
   f. gait evaluation and training.
5. The doctor is the patient's most important ally. If it appears that Medicare coverage will be denied, ask the doctor to help demonstrate that the standards described above are met.

6. If the nursing home informs the patient that Medicare coverage will terminate before the 100 days and the patient seems to satisfy the criteria above, ask the home to submit a claim for a formal Medicare determination. The nursing home must submit a claim if the patient or representative requests; the patient is not required to pay until s/he receives a formal determination from Medicare.
7. Don't be satisfied with a Medicare determination unreasonably limiting coverage; appeal for the benefits the patient deserves. It will take some time, but most appeals win. Appeal when you are right since if you lose the patient must pay the bill.

For more information on the law relating to the skilled care benefit see "Selected Medicare Regulations on Skilled Care"at the end of the book. For more information on preparation see our "Prepare Your Case for Review" comments in the **"Post Hospital Care"** section.

How to Appeal Premature Termination of the Medicare Skilled Benefit
Often the patient advocate is given information such as "rehab will end Friday" - rehabilitative therapy being the most commonly used Medicare skilled benefit. An oral communication is not sufficient for you to take *legal* action. You *must* receive *notice in writing.* Demand your proper notice and once you do you can begin the process by contacting KEPRO, (855) 408-8557, for an immediate review. They will issue their determination within 36 hours. If not favorable you should receive the written notice and then sign the request for appeal. You then follow the appeal steps in the notice. A hearing will be scheduled and you may have an attorney. In most cases the cost of care may make this step an unaffordable gamble, since Medicare appeals are for *reimbursement of incurred expense.*

Before you pursue your *legal* options review your advocacy options. How to respond to the information? Decide if you agree. The first point to consider if the patient is trying? If not, see if you can work out a plan. Having a family member present during therapy to encourage participation can produce results. Is the resident sleepy during therapy? Perhaps therapy should be scheduled for the patient's best time of day. For some it is morning and others it is the afternoon. Is the resident in too much pain? Maybe the therapy and pain medication need to be better coordinated. Try to determine the problem and a solution. Is the patient not trying because she is depressed? Perhaps medication for depression might work. Maybe a family member could be present to cheer and encourage her on. However, if he patient merely does not want to try then there is no point in continuation.

Is the reason for termination that the initial goal for therapy has been met? Should it be revised? What if the goal was that the patient would walk with a walker? What if the patient has made rapid progress, but not enough to return home and live independently? He may be able to walk with a walker but not able to manage the stairs in the home. If so, then the goal should be updated.

What if the reason is that the patient cannot make any more progress? What if you just *know* that more can be expected? Here we are considering the continuation *rehabilitative* therapy not *maintenance* therapy. Has the staff really observed progress made? Many times progress is slow, barely observable to those who do not know the patient. Is the patient functioning at her highest practical level? What if she broke her hip and can now walk with a walker, but cannot transfer from chair to walker? Do you think she could transfer if therapy were continued? Remember the Medicare benefit is to be used to achieve the highest practicable level of functioning.

Ideally you should not get to the point of appeal. As patient advocate you will have monitored your resident's progress under care you have "supervised." When skilled coverage is terminated you should be in agreement that no more benefit can be received. Nonetheless it is true that not all providers do the job they should.

If you cannot work out a continuation with the staff, prepare for the next step, the review by KEPRO, (855) 408-8557, the Medicare QIO. Be sure to have your facts. It is simply necessary to have the support of the patient's doctor. That is another a good reason to keep the patient under the treatment of her personal physician. Review will be completed in 24 to 48 hours.

The next step is formal appeal. Note, appeal does not continue Medicare payment. Medicare *payments* are ended until and unless reinstated by the judge on appeal. The patient must either pay for skilled care and look for reimbursement or incur the liability with the hope that Medicare will pay after appeal (where successful). Skilled care is very expensive and that is why you should take all steps to ensure success. Though the Medicare appeals are more "customer" friendly than courts, an attorney can be of key importance especially where the value of the benefits greatly exceeds the cost of the attorney.

If upon conclusion of Medicare skilled benefits the patient does not leave the nursing home the patient advocate will be presented with a contract by the nursing home. It may not require the signing of a contract as long as the patient is receiving those Medicare benefits. Contracts are covered in later sections.

The Medicare Hospice Benefit

Hospice is commonly understood as end of life care. While that part is true, hospice is much more. The essence of hospice is an alternate healthcare practice of palliative care. That means the focus is not on curing the condition but making the patient more comfortable. The Medicare benefit does not require a patient to be at end of life. In fact the Medicare requirement is that a doctor need only certify that death is reasonably likely within *six months*. Hospice is a Medicare benefit for alternative treatment. It is true that many people leave hospice because their health has improved. Medicare allows a person to elect hospice and elect out of hospice at will.

For those who qualify, hospice is an additional option on discharge. The information below is from the Centers for Medicare & Medicaid Services publication "*Medicare Hospice Benefits.*":

What is Hospice?
Hospice is a special way of caring for people who are terminally ill, and for their families. This care includes physical care and counseling. The goal of hospice is to care for you and your family, not to cure your illness. It is also a special Medicare benefit and may be an additional health insurance benefit.

Medicare covers hospice care if:
* You are eligible for Medicare Part A; and
* Your doctor and the hospice medical director certify that you are terminally ill and probably have less than six months to live; and
* You sign a statement choosing hospice care instead of routine Medicare covered benefits for your terminal illness; and
* You get care from a Medicare-approved hospice program.

Under your Medicare benefit you choose hospice as your treatment for the terminal condition. Medicare will still pay for covered benefits for <u>any</u> health problems that aren't related to your terminal illness. For example, a patient may enter a hospice program and still have her HMO Medicare provider handle claims for all other conditions.

If you qualify for hospice care, you will have a specially trained medical team and support staff available to help you and your family cope with your illness. Hospice comfort care helps you make the most of the last months of life. Hospice comfort care includes use of drugs for symptom control and pain relief, physical care, counseling, equipment, and supplies to make you as comfortable and pain free as possible. The focus of hospice is on care, not cure. Those involved in your care include:

- you, your family,
- a doctor, a nurse,
- counselors, a social worker,
- speech-language therapists,
- home health aides, homemakers, and volunteers.

What will Medicare pay for?
The care you get for your terminal illness must be from a Medicare-approved hospice program. You can receive a one-time-only hospice consultation with a hospice medical director or hospice physician to discuss your care options and management of pain and symptoms. You don't need to choose hospice care to take advantage of this consultation service. Medicare pays for these hospice services for your terminal illness and related conditions:
- Doctor services
- Nursing care
- Medical equipment (such as wheelchairs or walkers)
- Medical supplies (such as bandages and catheters)
- Drugs for symptom control or pain relief (you may need to pay a small co-payment)
- Home health aide and homemaker services
- Physical, occupational therapy and speech therapy
- Social worker services
- Dietary counseling
- Grief and loss counseling for you and your family
- Short-term inpatient care
- Short-term respite care (you may need to pay a small co-payment)
- Any other covered Medicare services needed to manage your pain and other symptoms, as recommended by your hospice team

What Is Respite Care?
Respite care is care given to a hospice patient by another caregiver so that the usual caregiver can rest. While in hospice care you may have one person who takes care of you every day, such as a family member. Sometimes this person needs someone to take care of you for a short time when he or she needs a break from care giving. During a period of respite care, you will be cared for in a Medicare-approved facility, such as a hospice inpatient facility, hospital, or nursing home.

Room and Board
Room and board is not a Medicare hospice benefit even if your receive the benefit in a nursing home or a hospice residential facility. However, if the hospice medical team determines that you need short-term inpatient or respite services that they arrange, your stay in the facility is covered. You may be required to pay a small co-payment for the respite stay.

Important: Hospice care is given in periods of care. You can get hospice care for two 90-day periods followed by an unlimited number of 60-day periods. At the start of each period of care, the hospice medical director or other hospice doctor must re-certify that you are terminally ill, so that you may continue to get hospice care. A period of care starts the day you begin to get hospice care. It ends when your 90-day or 60-day period ends.

Hospice Residence
While most people receive hospice care in their current residence be that home, assisted living or nursing home, there are hospice residences. Payment for these may be by private insurance or by **Medicaid** if the hospice has beds that are certified for hospice payment. Ask the residential provider about what they accept for payment for *all* charges.

Special Note: Check Your Insurance Coverage
Some pension plans have insurance that covers hospice over and above Medicare. Check your benefits booklet or your "Summary Plan Description" to learn what the your coverage includes. It may pay daily charges in a residential hospice.

A copy of the above publication is available at: www.medicare.gov/Pubs/pdf/02154.pdf

Managing Care In a Nursing Home
(You Can Get Good Care in a Nursing Home)

How does one get good care in a nursing home? The answer goes beyond selecting the right home. The patient or "resident" must have a patient advocate who will monitor the patient's condition by frequent visitation and communication with the nursing home staff. The advocate will ask questions, report problems and see that they are addressed. Many of the same strategies that you use to maximize your Medicare benefit can be used to get the best long term care.

Contrary to common belief, the nursing home is not a place to be passive about receiving care. Good care, including medical and personal, comes through patient advocacy by an informed, involved advocate. How does one do that? Families find that the world of nursing homes is completely new to them. Some families have found a way to quick-start the process: hire a nurse care manager. See that section below. Whether you hire professional assistance or not, your first step is to be informed.

> **You are in charge. You have hired these people.**

The Care Plan
The law requires every resident of a nursing home have a care plan. This is the same process that was covered above under the Medicare skilled care benefit.

Even with a care plan, we can expect things will not go smoothly and in some cases it will not go well at all. Here again, you must be vigilant and carefully watch the resident's condition.

The Professional Care Manager
The patient advocate may hire a "Professional Care Manager" who can quickly get the advocate up to speed. This person may be a nurse, social worker or other professional. It is not necessary for every patient or family to hire independent services. However, many have found that a Professional Care Manager can educate them on the role of the patient advocate in the nursing home, the patient's current treatment regimen, what to expect, what to look out for and how to get the best result.

What can the care manager do? Conduct an assessment of the patient. This would include a review the medical record, consult with patient's physician and medical team and then report and recommend to the patient advocate. The care manager could also assist the advocate and attend care conferences. The result would be an informed, individualized patient treatment program upon admission and ongoing.

If the need arises after admission the patient advocate would have an accurate assessment of the problem and steps to take to resolve it.

What If There Are Problems?
There are times when, even in the best of nursing homes, a person's condition deteriorates. Sometimes this is the path of the disease process and other times due to inadequate care. What can you do if you suspect that your loved one is not being properly cared for? You should be vigilant, educated and protective. Working in advance, you should exercise the patient's right to choose medical providers. This includes not only treating physicians but what hospital your patient may be moved to. Note, the exception here is that if 911 is called in emergency they are limited to which emergency room they can take a person. In all other cases if the nursing home's default choice is not satisfactory, choose the hospital in advance. You have authority to reject one and select another. But, what if there is a problem with care?

Involve Staff. You can and should report your concern to the appropriate staff. Depending on the nature of the problem it may involve aides, nurses, Director of Nursing, administration, or the doctor. For example, "bed sores" can be the result of inadequate resident attention by aides. If that continues the resident can develop very serious skin ulcers that will require hospital care. If the problem is a medical one, discuss it with the Director of Nursing and the doctor's assistant. If it is serious and the treatment team cannot tell you what is wrong, insist that they involve a specialist and if they do not, consider making an appointment with a doctor yourself as the healthcare agent.

Remember that the patient has the right to select her own doctor. That may mean arranging transportation of the patient to the doctor. The patient's personal physician will order the care/treatment plan. The nursing home doctor supervises the nursing home and the delivery of care.

Be a Patient Advocate. Actively monitor your patient's condition. Don't rely on the assurances of staff. Review the medical chart. Be watchful for a loss of weight – an indicator of declining health. Monitor prescribed medications and inquire of the nurse and doctor if there are changes you do not know about. Be especially vigilant about psychiatric medications. Know the side effects, interactions with other medications and changes that may result. Elders, especially those in poor health, may not be able to process the medication resulting in toxicity and emergency treatment.

Check her mouth for oral hygiene and ears for proper care. Inspect her to make sure she is cleaned. If you question the quality of bathing, put a mark on her. Look for bed sores. If a wound is bandaged, write a date on the bandage. Consider doing the laundry. That way you will know if clothing is soaked or soiled. Take pictures of her if there has been an upsetting incident.

Dehydration and Malnutrition. Be vigilant and monitor your loved one's nutrition and hydration. Studies have shown that many patient health problems arise from malnourishment and dehydration. When there are problems it is often because aides do not have the time to help all residents with their eating and drinking needs at meal times and in-between as well. When you visit, check and see if she completes her meals. Check and see if she is thirsty or has taken her fluids. Is the water glass within her reach? If you see a pattern, do not wait until she starts losing weight or worse. By that time your loved one's health is in decline.

Dehydration and Low Electrolytes - Sodium and Potassium
Dehydration means more than merely being thirsty, it also includes electrolyte imbalance in a patient's blood. And, if there is a problem with the electrolytes there may be a problem with the level of "toxins" from medications. For example we may say one is dehydrated if her sodium or potassium levels are seriously low. Low sodium may cause a person to be lethargic or confused. Staff may say "That's just the dementia getting worse. It's to be expected." But low sodium is not caused by dementia - it causes dementia. Low potassium can cause muscle weakness and exercise intolerance and that can be a cause for failure in skilled care rehab. It can also cause hallucinations, which may be mistakenly treated by antipsychotic medications.

Dehydration can be a perverse result of treatment. Low potassium can be caused by antibiotics and diuretics. Low sodium may result from antipsychotic medications used to treat dementia patients who become aggressive or, as observed above, to treat confusion that is the result of low potassium. Failure to diagnose *this form of dehydration will lead to a worsening condition that can result in death. See Taking Charge: Good Medical Care for the Elderly and How to Get It* by Michigan attorney Jeanne M. Hannah and Joseph H. Friedman, M.D. (2006). Ms. Hannah tells the story how her mother went from an active 83 year old lady to dead in 65 days. Remember: **Dehydration can kill.**

Get Help. If you do not get immediate cooperation in resolving your concern, contact the State Long Term Care Ombudsman Office, a professional care manager or an elder law attorney such as the author. See the **Resources** section in the back of this book.

Good care is a combination of selecting the right home, knowing the patient's rights and regularly visiting and monitoring and managing your loved one's treatment. In other words, being a real "patient advocate."

Conclusion

Remember that there is a legal obligation between the nursing home and your loved one. In exchange for a monthly fee, the nursing home has agreed to provide individualized care to maintain the highest level of well-being for your loved one. In addition, the home is required by law to improve, or if not possible, maintain her health.

In your role as advocate you will be the vigilant protector. You will participate in the care planning forum to bring your information, questions and concerns to the table. You will identify your loved one's needs and develop solutions for any problems that may arise. You will monitor the delivery of care. In short, you are in charge of the treatment team.

The Nursing Home Contract
(You __do__ have rights)

Since no contract is required for Medicare skilled care, the patient advocate will not be presented with a nursing home contract as long as Medicare is paying the bill. But if the patient will remain in the nursing home at the end of Medicare skilled care, then a signed contract will be required. Of course, if the patient/resident enters the nursing home without a Medicare stay then the patient advocate will be presented with one upon admission. These contracts are regulated by law. There are limits to what the nursing home can demand.[2]

A note of caution: Yes, the patient/resident has rights. But, rights can be waived by the patient. They can also be waived by you, the patient advocate. Courts have approved waivers that are "hidden" in paragraphs of the multi-page contract. The fact that they are buried in pages of single space contract is no defense. The law presumes a person knows what he or she is signing. As the saying goes "ignorance of the law is no excuse." And we might adapt that to say "ignorance of the contract is no excuse." Now you as the patient advocate will be given a pile of papers to sign. Many are harmless and necessary paperwork. You should insist on time to read before you sign - maybe take them to the patient's room to review. Anything that is title "agreement" is a flag for a binding contract. You should have an elder law attorney review any "agreement" or contract before you sign.

On entry into long term care, the nursing home will provide an admission agreement or contract. The law requires nursing homes to provide detailed contracts with "residents." Nursing homes are licensed under section 21711 of the Public Health Code, *Michigan Compiled Laws* (MCL) 333.21711. The law and regulations that create rights in the home's residents also cover admission contracts.

Written Contract Required
The Michigan law regulating the contracts of admission to a nursing home is found at Michigan Compiled Laws (MCL) 333.21766. The contract must be written in "clear and unambiguous" language. *Id,* Section (6). The contract must specify all of the following:
    (a) The term of the contract.
    (b) The services to be provided under the contract and the charges for the services.
    (c) The services that may be provided to supplement the contract and the charges for the services.

---

2 You will notice below the references to "MCL, USC and CFR." These are used so that you know it is the law, not the author's opinion, and so you can look up the "citations" and the law yourself.

(d) The sources liable for payments due under the contract.

(e) The amount of deposit paid and the general and foreseeable terms upon which the deposit will be held and refunded.

(f) The rights, duties, and obligations of the patient, except that the specification of a patient's rights may be furnished on a separate document that complies with the requirements of section 20201 (the resident's rights section).

MCL 333.21766(7). The contract must specify all services and charges, including those not included in the per diem rate.

Required Financial Disclosure

As noted in (d) above, the admission contract must address the sources liable for payments. Michigan law further provides that a patient is responsible for providing the facility with "accurate and timely information concerning his or her sources of payment and ability to meet financial obligations." MCL 333.20202(7). This disclosure of financial ability does not create a guarantee that the resident will not apply for Medicaid within a set period of time or that the resident will spend the money on the nursing home. *See* "Illegal Admission Requirements."

Financial Admission Discrimination

May a facility use the financial disclosure information and discriminate against applicants who have less funds? There is no protection against it. The Nursing Home Reform Law does not address the issue. The law prohibits discrimination based on source of payment in ``transfer, discharge, and the provision of services.'' It does not address admissions. 42 United States Code (USC) 1396r (c)(4)(a) , 42 Code Federal Regulations (CFR) 483.12 (d)(1).

Illegal Admission Requirements

No Third Party Guarantee.
Federal law *prohibits* a *requirement* of a third-party guarantee of payment, 42 USC 1395i-3(c)(5)(A)(ii), 1396r(c)(5)(A)(ii); 42 CFR. Section 483.12(d)(2). However, a person may *voluntarily* agree to be responsible. *You must be careful to read the admission agreement so that you are not "tricked" into a "voluntary" guarantee.* Some nursing home contracts have language buried in the middle pages of the agreement where it says the person signing is responsible for payment and securing Medicaid. Be safe and have a lawyer review what you are given to sign.

A Patient Advocate May Not Be Required.
Michigan law does not allow a nursing home to require a patient advocate designation to be executed as a condition of providing, withholding, or withdrawing care, custody, or medical treatment. Federal law does not allow a home to condition the provision of care or otherwise discriminate against an individual based on whether or not the individual has executed an advance directive. 42 CFR 489.102(a)(3).

While a facility may not require an advance directive, it must inform all adult residents concerning the right to accept or refuse medical or surgical treatment and, at the individual's option, formulate an advance directive. 42 CFR 483.10 (b)(8).

A Guardian May Not be Required for admission.
Michigan's guardian statute requires consideration of less restrictive alternatives before a petition is filed. The petitioner must be informed of the alternatives including, but not limited to, a limited guardian, conservator, patient advocate designation, do-not-resuscitate declaration, or durable power of attorney with or without limitations on purpose, authority, or time period, and an explanation of each alternative. MCL 700.5303 (2).

No Minimum Payment before Applying for Medicaid.
A home certified for Medicaid may not require oral or written assurances that the resident will not apply for Medicaid. 42 USC 1396r(c)(5)(A)(ii), MCL 333.21765a(1).

Michigan law further prohibits a nursing home from requiring a patient to remain in private pay status for a specified period of time before applying for Medicaid. MCL 333.21765a(2). The law does not prohibit an inquiry of a patient about "accurate and timely information concerning his or her sources of payment and ability to meet financial obligations." MCL 333.20202(7). Contracts that go beyond disclosure and attempt to disallow "divestment" or require the applicant apply the assets disclosed to the nursing home bill violate Michigan and federal law.

A person who violates section MCL 333.21765a (1) or (2) is liable to an applicant or patient in a civil action for *treble* the amount of actual damages or $1,000.00, whichever is greater, together with costs and reasonable attorney fees. MCL 333.21799c(2).

No Required Deposit of Funds.
A contract may not require direct deposit of resident's income to the facility. 42 USC 1395i-3(c)(6)(A)(i), 1396r(c)(6)(A)(i); 42 CFR 483.10(c)(1). Nor may the home require the resident to turn over funds or property to the home. MCL 333.20201 (3)(g). However a resident may require the home to manage resident funds and hold them in a trust account. MCL 333.20201 (3)(c).

Consult with an Attorney
If you believe the contract/agreement has illegal provisions, or a staff person is making an illegal demand, see an attorney. You should also contact the Long Term Care Ombudsman at 866-485-9393.

The "Responsible Party"
Federal regulations and Michigan law allow an admission contract to provide for a designated "responsible party." That refers to a person with access to the resident's funds or assets. The responsible party does not incur personal financial obligation other than to use the resident's funds on behalf of the resident, MCL 333.21766(9). The "responsible party" may be required to provide facility payment from the *resident's* income or resources. 42 CFR 483.12 (d)(2). Michigan law require a person with access to a resident's funds, an agent or joint tenant for example, to be responsible for paying the nursing home bills *from the resident's funds*, MCL 333.21766(8).

Being a responsible party does not make one liable for the nursing home bill. It is illegal to require a "third party guarantee," *see above*. However if responsible party misappropriates the resident's funds then he or she may face criminal prosecution.

A responsible party *may* be found liable for the bill if he or she signs nursing home contract/agreement that includes language such as "the responsible party shall be responsible for obtaining Medicaid approval." Many admission agreements have such provisions. Before you sign the contract, have a lawyer review it. You can be certain the contract was written by the nursing home's lawyer for the benefit of the nursing home.

The above does not mean the patient's representative payee need not use the patient's funds for the patient's benefit, *including payment of the nursing home*. That would be illegal as elder abuse or criminal embezzlement.

The responsible party should exercise great caution if the resident does not have enough money for all bills. Suppose savings are running out: what bills should be paid? Should you pay the credit card off and not pay the nursing home? Should you pay the taxes on the home and not other bills? Can you prepay a funeral for the resident? If you are in this situation, seek legal counsel lest you be sued yourself.

Advocate's Tip: Have the Patient Sign the Admission Contract

Citizens who enter a nursing home does not lose their legal rights. They have the right to be treated as adults who can make their own legal agreements. A patient advocate, whether spouse, child, sibling or friend is under no duty to sign a nursing home contract. That is true even if the person is the patient's representative payee for social security funds. So, if you signed the agreement go back to the admission office and say the resident wants to sign her own agreement. Get a new agreement/contract, have her sign and then have the admission person tear up the one you signed.

A helpful person who is assisting the patient can avoid being sued on the contract by simply refusing to sign. This refusal could lead to refusal of *admission* to an applicant, but it cannot lead to *discharge* of a patient who already has a bed. For example, upon completion of the Medicare paid skilled care many facilities approach the patient advocate with a contract to sign as "responsible party." What if neither the patient nor the patient advocate sign the contact? The facility may not discharge a resident because the contract was not signed. However, contract terms would still apply to the resident but not to the patient advocate.

Note that if the patient and advocate do not cooperate for legal reasons, nursing home may file for probate guardianship claiming that they are interfering with care of the patient. Advocating for the patient's best care and protection of rights is not grounds for the appointment of a probate guardian. But obstructing care for a patient/resident can be grounds for the probate court to appoint a guardian.

Under the law a patient that is not able to make informed medical decisions may have a probate guardian appointed for him or her. If family members are not acting in the patient's best interest a probate guardian may be appointed. If the nursing home files the guardian petition in probate court they will ask for an attorney or guardian company to be appointed. Nursing homes are familiar with these professionals who are often cooperative. While the patient advocate may ask to be appointed guardian at the court hearing, the judge may refuse.

In short, it is better to work with the Long Term Care Ombudsman and hire an attorney to work out any dispute with the nursing home before matters end up in the probate court.

Nursing Home Residents' Rights
(Residents have rights and you don't have to pay their bill)

The source of the rights of nursing home residents is the law Congress passed in 1987 to address the serious problems of care in nursing homes. The law is known as the "Nursing Home Reform Law." Since it was passed as part of that year's budget bill, the Omnibus Budget Reconciliation Act, it is also known as OBRA 87. This law applies to nursing homes that participate in the Medicare or Medicaid program. Michigan followed federal law and passed a law protecting nursing home patients rights. It is found in *Michigan Compiled Laws* (MCL) 333.20201(2), (3). It applies to all nursing homes. The resident's rights guaranteed by federal law are found in the *United States Code* (USC) and the *Code of Federal Regulations* (CFR). Not all and every nuance are included here. Some of the major rights follow.

The Right to Achieve and Maintain the Highest Practicable Level of Functioning
Some patients are critically ill or "actively dying." Others are long term residents. All residents have the right to maintain function not affected by their illness. The resident has the right to, and the nursing home must provide services, including:
- therapy (physical, speech and occupational). For example, it is a violation of a resident's right to cause a loss of ability to walk where the loss is not a necessary result of the patient's medical condition;
- assistance with Activities of Daily Living (ADL) – eating, bathing, grooming, transferring and ambulating.

Given the wide spread problem of malnutrition and dehydration, reported by the Commonwealth Fund and others, it is hard to overstate the importance of assistance with ADLs to maintain independence. The advocate can find provisions in 42 USC 1396r(b)(4)(A)(I), the statute, and 42 CFR 483.45, the regulation that require these needs be met in the residents plan of care.

The Right to Make Health Care Decisions
Federal law, 42 USC 1396r(c)(1)(A)(i), 42 C.F.R, Section 483.10(b)(4), guarantees the right to:
- make medical treatment decisions, unless judged incompetent;
- decide who the attending physician will be;
- accept or refuse medical treatment;
- be fully informed in advance of any changes in care or treatment that may affect the resident's well being;
- the right to review and have copies of medical records;
- participate in planning care and treatment or changes in care and treatment by the patient or advocate.

The right to make health care decisions and participate in the process is fundamental to the concept of quality care in a nursing home through patient rights.

The Right to Be Free of Unnecessary Restraints

Physical or medical restraints not required to treat the resident's condition are not allowed. A restraint may be imposed only upon a physician's order <u>and</u> the patient or advocate's agreement. 42 USC 1396r(c)(1)(A)(ii).

The Right to Be Free From Abuse

The resident has the right to be free of willful abuse be it physical or mental. Abuse encompasses intimidation or punishment resulting in harm or anguish.

The Right to Accommodation of Individual Needs and Preferences

The nursing home must allow the resident to choose "activities, schedules, and health care consistent with his or her interests, assessments and plans of care." 42 CFR 483.15(b). The only exception is health and safety of the residents.

The Right to Independence, Dignity and Participation in All Activities.

The patient's right to dignity and independence is stated by the right to:
- privacy in treatment, communications and visits with family. 1396r(c)(1)(A)(iii).
- confidentiality of records. 1396r(c)(1)(A)(iv).
- have grievances addressed by the facility. 1396r(c)(1)(A)(vi).
- participate in resident or family groups. 1396r(c)(1)(A)(vii).
- participate in social, religious or community groups. 1396r(c)(1)(A)(viii).
- examine survey reports made by the state or federal inspectors.

See also a comparable list under 42 USC. 1395i-3(c)(1)(A)(i).

No Waiver of Rights.

A nursing home may not require individuals applying to reside or residing in the facility to waive their rights. 42 USC 1395i-3(c)(5)(A)(ii), 1396r(c)(5)(A)(ii).

Getting Help: The Long Term Care Ombudsman

You can get authoritative assistance from the Michigan Long Term Care Ombudsman is an independent agency. Their phone number is **1-866-485-9393.** Their web address is http://mltcop.org/

Their mission statement:

> "The Michigan Long-Term Care Ombudsman program was created to help address the quality of care experienced by residents living in licensed long-term care facilities such as nursing homes, homes for the aged, and adult foster care facilities."

Summary

Congress recognized the rights of nursing home residents to quality care in the nursing home. These rights are not obstructions to good care but the guarantee of it. If the rights are observed the patient will have individualized care with maximum respect for the patient's person, independence and dignity.

The Six and Only Reasons for Discharge

A nursing home may inform you of its intention to discharge your family member. This commonly happens when he or she is difficult to care for and especially true if "agitated" and upsetting other residents. It happens when Medicaid drags its feet and the home has not been paid for months. It happens when Medicaid denies an application. Can the nursing home effect an involuntary discharge in times like these?

These are the *only* reasons the law allows an involuntary discharge of a resident. A nursing home may involuntarily discharge a patient when:

    (1) transfer or discharge is necessary for the resident's welfare because the resident's needs cannot be met in a nursing facility;

    (2) transfer or discharge is appropriate because the resident's health has improved to the point that s/he no longer needs nursing facility services;

    (3) the resident's presence endangers the safety of individuals in the facility;

    (4) the resident's presence endangers the health of individuals in the facility;

    (5) the resident has failed to pay (or to have paid under Medicare or Medicaid) for facility services; or

    (6) the facility is going out of business.

42 USC 1396r(c)(2)(A), 42 CFR 483.12. Michigan follows federal law, MCL 333.21773. Note that (5) is satisfied if If a resident has submitted appropriate paperwork to a third party payer and is waiting for a response to the claim. That paperwork may be a Medicaid application or the filing a claim with your insurance carrier.

The discharge notice must be written and be given a minimum of 30 days before the proposed discharge. The 30 day requirement may be waived if medically necessary as shown by written orders and medical justification of the attending physician, or if mandated by the physical safety of other patients and facility employees. The notice must be accompanied by notice of the right to appeal. MCL 333.21773.

Appeal of Discharge

Upon receipt of a Notice of an Involuntary Transfer or Discharge to a nursing home resident, the resident or authorized representative may file an appeal with the Department of Community Health. This appeal must be in writing and made within ten days of the date of the notice to the Director of the Department. A Request for Hearing will then be sent to the Bureau of Hearings who will notify you of the hearing date to be held at the facility. For more information see https://www.michigan.gov/documents/mdch/bhs_GUIDANCE_for_Inv_Transfer_32182 0_7.pdf

Planning Prior to Discharge

A nursing home is strictly limited in discharge procedures. They may not simply "put him in the lobby" and tell the family to "come and get him." Whenever a home discharges a patient, voluntary or involuntary, it must have a discharge plan that will meet the patient's needs.

The patient may disagree with the discharge plan, file a complaint and have a hearing on the adequacy of the plan. Your first action should be to contact the Long Term Care Ombudsman (below) as soon as you hear of the discharge plan, and if discharge notice has been given then ask for a review of the discharge plan by **KEPRO, (855) 408-8557**.

A complaint may be made by the Complaint Hotline (800) 882-6006 or online at: www6.dleg.state.mi.us/parsers/complaints/onlineform.asp

Note: Transfer to Hospital is <u>Not</u> Discharge

There are times when a nursing home will transfer a difficult patient to the hospital for treatment. The patient is <u>not</u> discharged, even if the patient does not pay a bed hold fee. Often the facility will not have a vacant bed when the patient is discharged from the hospital. What then? The hospital discharge planner must make another nursing home placement. That does <u>not</u> mean the patient has been discharged from the first nursing home. The patient has the right to return to the facility to the first available bed.

If the nursing home wants to discharge a patient the home *must follow formal discharge procedures* including 30 day notice and information of the right to appeal. Once a person is admitted as a resident s/he may only be discharged for one of the six reasons above. The burden of proof is *very* high. The facility is in the business of meeting the medical needs of its residents. To discharge it must show that the particular condition is not one that it is licensed to treat, a difficult proof to make.

The Long Term Care Ombudsman

If the patient or advocate has any complaint with the patient's treatment or a violation of the patient's rights they may ask the Michigan Long Term Care Ombudsman for help. Call 1-866-485-9393. See the "Resources" section for more.

The Long Term Care Ombudsman office is required by Federal and Michigan law. The Ombudsman duties are to identify, investigate, and resolve complaints made by residents regarding the health, safety, welfare, or rights of the residents (including the welfare and rights of the residents with respect to the appointment and activities of guardians and representative payees). The Ombudsman will also represent the interests of the resident before governmental agencies and seek administrative, legal, and other remedies to protect the health, safety, welfare, and rights of the residents. The Ombudsman program is established in federal law found at 42 USC 3058g and Michigan statute at MCL 400.586h.

Medicaid – Payment for Long Term Care
(Pay the Nursing Home Without Going Broke)

Many people think Medicare will pay for the nursing home. It does not pay for long term care. It only has a limited post-hospital nursing home benefit for "skilled care." The *maximum* benefit is 100 days. While it's never possible to predict at the outset how long Medicare approve payment for skilled care, from our experience it often falls far short of the 100 day maximum. If Medicare does cover the 100 day period, what then? Unless the patient has supplemental skilled care insurance, the patient will have to pay by long term care insurance, life savings, or apply for Medicaid.

Medicare is the program that all wage earners and dependants over 65 receive. Its benefits are very limited in the nursing home. Medicare only pays for "skilled care" up to 100 days. It does not pay for long term care. Medicare does not pay for nursing home care for all diseases or conditions that result in long term care, for example Alzheimer's or Parkinson's disease. Even though the patient receives medical care, it is not *skilled care.* Of course if such patient needs skilled care, such after surgery for a broken hip, Medicare will pay for that. Medicaid will pay for long term care in a nursing home, if the resident applies and is eligible.

Those who do not enter the nursing home on a Medicare stay are must arrange payment from other sources, right from the start. The options are: 1) long term care insurance; 2) "private pay" out of life-savings; 3) Medicaid if an application is made for the benefit and is approved.

What is Medicaid?
Medicaid is a long term care program you have already paid for by your taxes. It is "means tested." Medicaid is overseen by the Centers for Medicare and Medicaid Services (CMS). It is primarily funded by the federal government, the states fund the remainder and administer the program. In Michigan the agency is the Department of Health and Human Services.

One must apply for Medicaid and prove "eligibility." It is a complicated, at times illogical, benefits program drafted by Congress, implemented by states with variations in program and interpretation. That means rules do vary from state to state. Sometimes application of "policy" varies from county to county in a state.

How Does Medicaid Work?
Medicaid will pay for nursing home care if the applicant:
    1) the patient needs nursing home level of care;
    2) if the patient is financially eligible;
    3) is in a Medicaid bed;

4) has no "divestment penalty period;"

5) successfully completes an application.

All of the above steps must be satisfied. And finally we will add a sixth item of Medicaid and that is:

6) post-death estate recovery. The government comes after your home.

Problems with all of the above can be avoided with competent advice and representation.

The complexities and lack of knowledge about Medicaid make professional advice essential to avoid a substantial loss of money and property. Even the family home is at risk. We consider each below.

The Requirements for a Successful Medicaid Application

Requirement 1: "Seven Doors to Medicaid"
An applicant must need a level of care severe enough to require nursing home care. Medicaid uses the "Seven Doors" screen to make that determination. One will satisfy the proof of need for a nursing home by meeting the standards of any one of the "doors." The doors or screens are:

1. **Activities of Daily Living**. The patient needs supervision or extensive assistance with moving around in bed, transferring from bed to chair or wheelchair, or standing, toileting or eating.

2. **Cognitive Performance**. The patient has severe problems with memory or making decisions about basic daily needs.

3. **Physician Involvement**. The patient is under the care of a physician for treatment of an unstable medical condition.

4. **Treatments and Conditions**. The patient has received treatment for conditions in the last two weeks: diabetes with daily insulin and order changes; stage 3-4 pressure sores; intravenous or parenteral feedings; intravenous medications; end of life care (life expectancy less than 6 months); daily tracheostomy care, daily respiratory care, daily suctioning, pneumonia, daily oxygen therapy, peritoneal or hemodialysis.

5. **Skilled Rehabilitation Therapies**. Has the patient been scheduled to receive, or is receiving, speech, occupational, or physical therapies and continues to require skilled rehabilitation therapies?

6. **Behaviors**. Wandering, verbal or physical abuse, socially inappropriate behavior, resists care, hallucinations or delusions.

7. **Service Dependency**. The patient has been a Medicaid participant for at least one year and requires ongoing services to maintain current functional status. No other community, residential or informal services are available to meet the patients needs.

We have reprinted the Seven Doors to Medicaid at the end of this book.

Fail the Seven Doors Screen?
Failure to pass any of the screens means that the person does not need nursing home care. What should the Patient Advocate do? Before you reconsider a re-assessment of the person's need you should be sure that the screen was not based on inaccurate or incomplete information. Speak with whomever did the screen. Review the screening *and* the medical chart of the patient before asking for a second screen. Make sure all care needs are recognized and recorded. Do your own screen using the 7 Doors To Medicaid in the back of this book. You may request a re-screening at any time. It may be requested the same day as the first screening. Once the 7 Doors screen is accurately done your patient's needs will be recognized.

If you agree your patient/resident does not pass the 7 Doors screen, that means he or she does not need a nursing home. You need a good individualized discharge plan. For example, the resident may not be able to return to home because there is no one who can assist and the resident cannot afford in-home care. Note that even if the resident fails the 7 Doors screen, he may still qualify for the "MiChoice Waiver" Medicaid program. It might pay for enough care for the resident to leave the nursing to home or an assisted living facility. Contact the local Area Agency on Aging about application procedures and to determine their waiting list.

The VA improved pension program should be considered if the resident is a wartime veteran or surviving spouse of such a veteran. This VA program provides a monthly cash benefit to help with "unreimbursed medical expenses" such as paying for help with Activities of Daily Living.

Requirement 2: Applicant Must be Financially Eligible

Medicaid will pay for nursing home care if the applicant is "resource eligible." Medicaid breaks financial resources into two categories: income and assets. To qualify for Medicaid the applicant must *not* have sufficient *income* to pay the medical bills. This is not a problem in the nursing home. The applicant is strictly limited in the amount and kind of *assets* that may be kept. Each category has its own rules.

The applicant will be eligible if she meets the asset test, that is she must not have excess "countable assets." Before we get into that, let's first understand what "assets" are.

Excluded Assets and Countable Assets

The main categories of Medicaid assets are *"excluded"* and *"countable"* assets. *Excluded assets* are those which Medicaid will not take into account at the time of application. The primary excluded assets are:

- Homestead, equity limited to $552,000 if no spouse. The home must have been the principal place of residence and the nursing home resident must "intend to return home" even if this never actually takes place. The limit is removed if a spouse, child under 21, or the client's blind or disabled child is residing in the home.
- Ordinary and usual personal belongings and household goods
- One vehicle
- Equity in income-producing real estate, equity limited to $6,000.
- Burial spaces and certain related items for applicant, spouse and immediate family members
- Up to $1,500 designated as a burial fund for applicant and spouse
- Irrevocable prepaid funeral contract
- Life insurance of face value $1,500 or less.

- Assets that applicant or spouse do not have the legal right to use or dispose of are excluded from countable assets.

- Real Estate that has been for sale for at least thirty days during the last three months and has not been sold. The asking price must be at fair market value and no asking price purchase offer may have been denied.

Most other assets are *countable* and subject to "spend down." Essentially all money and property, and any item that can be valued and turned into cash, is a countable asset unless it is one of those assets listed above as excluded. This includes:

A. Money in:
- Cash, savings and checking accounts, credit union share and draft accounts
- Certificates of deposit
- U.S. Savings Bonds
- Individual retirement accounts (IRA), Keogh plans, (401Ks, 403Bs)
- Nursing home trust funds
- Prepaid funeral contracts which can be canceled
- Trusts (depending on the terms of the trust)

B. Equity in:
- Real estate
- second motor vehicle, boats or recreational vehicles
- Stocks, bonds and mutual funds
- Land contracts or mortgages held on real estate sold

While the Medicaid rules themselves are complicated and tricky, it's safe to say that a single person will *not* qualify for Medicaid until the "countable assets" are $2,000 or less. That does mean Medicaid will not pay one penny if you have $2,001.

Medicaid "Spend Down"

The applicant must have no more than the maximum allowable "countable assets." The process of reducing the amount of such assets is called "spend down." Here are common examples of spend down:

- Pay Bills. Medicaid does not allow a credit for outstanding bills. For example a person may have $5,000 in the bank and owe $25,000 on the home mortgage. Medicaid would be denied until the $5,000 is spent down to $2,000. Sometimes there is not enough money for all bills. In that case talk to an elder law attorney about which to pay.

- Prepaid Funeral. Medicaid regulations permit the purchase of a prepaid funeral within limits. See your elder law attorney or reputable funeral director for guidance.

- Home Purchase. A community spouse may purchase a new home, even after the applicant enters the nursing home and it will be excluded. Where there is no spouse, the applicant may not purchase a home after long term care entry.

- Home Repair/maintenance. Money may be spent on needed maintenance or repairs, but they must be done quickly to be spent down.

- Home Improvements. Expenditures on the home are not limited to repairs. You can make improvements as well. But be sure you are not improving it just for the State of Michigan. See Requirement 6 below.

- New Car. One might consider purchasing a new car, though it is a declining investment.

- Long-Term Care Insurance for a Healthy Spouse. While long term care insurance will not be available for the nursing home resident the at home spouse may qualify.

Advanced Strategies. There are a number of advanced strategies that can reduce countable assets without "spending." These depend on the applicant's specific situation. An experienced Medicaid planning or elder law attorney should be consulted. If the attorney is not experienced you can lose thousands of dollars while the attorney "gets up to speed" on your case.

Requirement 3: Applicant must Be in a Medicaid Bed
Medicaid will not pay a nursing home bill unless the applicant is in a "Medicaid bed." Without the "Medicaid bed," Medicaid will not pay even if the person spent down and was approved for Medicaid. For most nursing homes this is not a problem. It is a problem in nursing homes that try to limit the number of long term care residents in favor of serving the post hospital Medicare skilled patients. See the tables in the back of the book to see if your nursing home is only "partially certified" for Medicaid. No Medicaid bed means transfer to a nursing home that does have an open Medicaid bed. That is why when you believe it will be long term care be sure that discharge from a hospital is to a home that has 100% Medicaid certification. See our list of nursing homes in the back of the book.

Requirement 4: Applicant Must Not have a Divestment Penalty
Since February 8, 2006, when President Bush signed the Deficit Reduction Act of 2005, Medicaid has a <u>five year look back</u>. Before then it was three years and some people still remember that. The look back means that an applicant must disclose all transfers of assets within the five years before the date of application.

"Divestment" refers to the act of divesting oneself of assets to get down to financial eligibility. It is broader than giving away assets. It includes purchasing assets for more than "fair market value." Divestment includes not only gifts but any action that reduces the applicants control over an asset. It includes adding names property, removing names from accounts and more. For example adding co-owners to real estate or investment accounts can be divestment since the co-owners now own part of the property. Some transfers are permitted such as those between husband and wife.

Divestment made within the look back period will be treated as though being made *when the person applies for Medicaid,* which could be up to five years later.

Divestment creates "penalty period." That is a period of time during which Medicaid will not pay the nursing home. This period will *only after application for Medicaid* and the person is in a nursing home. Divestment as small $276 will result in a one day penalty period. Greater amounts result in longer periods.

> Example: Within five years of applying for Medicaid, Mrs. King "loaned" her son $15,000 to avoid foreclosure on his home and gave two grandchildren a gift of $1,000 on their graduation. None of this money can be returned to her. Result: Total "transfers" of $17,000. A penalty period over two months will begin *after* she has applied and after she has spent down to $2,000. How she will pay during the two month penalty period when she has only $2,000 is unknown.

Requirement 5: Applicant Must Successfully Complete the Application Process
Here are the necessary minimum conditions for a successful application:

1. Be sure you have authority to apply for the nursing home resident. Unless you have a power of attorney that authorizes application for government benefits, you may have to be petition the probate court to be appointed the resident's guardian and conservator. When it comes to maximizing the savings allowed by Medicaid's "loopholes" probate court can be both unfriendly, slow and very expensive.

2. Get a copy of the Medicaid application and be sure you have written proof for everything you write down. Failure to provide adequate documentation will result in dismissal of the application. It absolutely must be complete.

3. Prepare to report any transfer of assets including closing of an account and putting the proceeds in another. Tax returns and bank accounts should be investigated for missing assets. Be sure you have *all* assets. Check safe deposit boxes, look for CDs and insurance policies. Inquire of siblings about assets. Sometimes a parent will buy a car for a child and not tell the others. Inquire about loans or gifts. These will be considered divestment. If assets have been "divested" see an experienced elder law attorney.

4. Plan to Apply Timely. Ordinarily an application should be filed as soon as spend down is complete. But planning for the application and spend down must begin as

soon as long term care is certain. Application processing by the Department of Human Services often takes months. If it is denied there may not be time to correct the mistake and get full coverage. However, an application will simply be denied if filed before spend down is complete. That means have your spend down and documentation of assets and expenditures well organized. In a rare case an application can be filed too early if a substantial divestment must be reported and the five years has almost run on the transfer of assets. In that case better to wait until the five years has run and then file the application.

5. Remember, it is a process. It is not enough to file a complete application. You must be able to give the Medicaid worker information requested in the short period of time allowed. For example you will need current values of all assets and those must be in writing. You must be able to document your spend down and the closing of accounts. Be prepared. Be on alert for the request to come by mail to you, your resident's home or to the nursing home. You do have the right to ask for one extension of 10 days, but that may not be enough time for you to get the information requested. Your application will be denied, you will have to reapply and you may lose months of coverage. The nursing home may sue to recover the unpaid bills.

Requirement 6: Plan for Post-death Estate Recovery
The government wants pay-back after the death of the Medicaid recipient. Under the current Michigan program this is done through probate. That means that any legal work done for Medicaid eligibility should contemplate probate avoidance as well. The state collection office will contact the family after the recipient has died, whether or not probate will be commenced. You should contact an elder law attorney upon receipt of the notice.
If probate is needed, the state will present its reimbursement claim. Note that the probate process and the estate recovery program have allowances, deductions and credits. It is best to contact an elder law attorney in this case.

Should I Seek Professional Advice for Medicaid?
Yes. Consider the income tax return. Most elders have their return done by a professional. Why? To be sure to save as much as possible. You will find that if you hire an elder law attorney you will save much, much more than any fee charged. As we have discussed above, the Medicaid application process is much more complex than any income tax return. That correctly implies that a professional offers three advantages: first, you will be advised of "loopholes" you did not know about; second, your application will be completed quicker than you could have which means earlier Medicaid coverage; and three, the application process will be successfully completed without denial. And, we might add a fourth: If you make a mistake in the application process, it is *your* mistake. If an attorney makes the mistake, it is the *attorney's* mistake.

Consider what is at risk - the average cost of a nursing home in Michigan is $8,282 per month. The applicant will get only one chance on application – it will be approved or denied. The needs and security of the patient and family is at stake. Without professional assistance many people find their application is needlessly, legitimately and avoidably denied. Mistakes are extremely expensive. The family security is irreversibly damaged.

So the answer is "Yes, immediately get advice" whether the applicant has little or much that must be "spent down." If nothing else use a bit of the spend down on attorney review the application you propose to submit. It will be inexpensive insurance against denial of benefits.

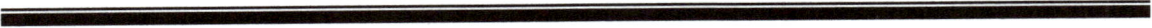

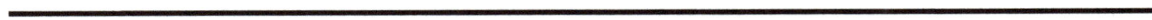

Medicaid – Questions & Misconceptions

"Do they count joint accounts with someone other than my spouse?"
Yes. The entire amount is counted unless the applicant can prove some of the money belongs to the other person. This rule applies to cash assets such as:

- Savings and checking accounts
- Credit union share and draft accounts
- Certificates of deposit
- U.S. Savings Bonds

"Can I give my assets or income away?"
Giving away or *divesting* assets or income for less than fair market value by the applicant, spouse or joint owner will result in a penalty period. "Divestment" includes:

- allowing another person to take assets or income from a joint account, and
- losing control over an asset by adding a joint owner or putting the property in certain kinds of trusts.

Divestment of assets during the look back period will result in a "penalty period." That means Medicaid will not pay the nursing home bill for period that is determined by the amount of the assets divested. Medicaid looks at transfers that occur up to five years before application for nursing home.   However, there is no penalty if assets are transferred in accordance with the Medicaid rules between spouses, to blind or disabled children, or are transfers for value.

"I heard I can give away $14,000 per year. Can't I?"
Many people have heard of the *federal Gift Tax* provision that allows them to give away $14,000 per year. What they do not know is that this refers to a Gift Tax exemption. It is not an absolute right. You may give away $14,000 per year per person without incurring tax, but those gifts will result in months of Medicaid ineligibility.

Still, some parents want to make gifts to their children before their life-savings are all gone. There are limited circumstances when assets may be transferred to others within the look-back period. In addition there is a Medicaid asset protection strategy that uses gifts to children. These rules are subject to change and you should consult with an elder law attorney if gifts or transfers have been or will be made during the five year look-back period.

Myth: Medicaid Will Not Provide Quality Care
Many people are concerned that if they have Medicaid pay the nursing home bills, they must go without quality healthcare. That is false. Almost all nursing homes are "Medicaid" nursing homes. An inspection of the nursing home listings in the back

of this book will show that few homes in Michigan do not participate in Medicaid. What if Medicaid does not cover a treatment? You can still get uncovered medical services paid, see below.

Do I Lose My Other Insurance If I Receive Medicaid Assistance?

No. Medicaid allows and one might say encourages medical insurance such as Blue Cross. The Medicaid recipient's "monthly patient pay amount" is the amount the patient must pay to the nursing home each month from his monthly income. Not all of the income goes to the nursing home. Medicaid allows a deduction for monthly health insurance premiums. Patients keep their private insurance and Medicaid covers the rest.

Medicaid Tip: Purchase Additional Insurance

A too little known provision is that Medicaid will allow a patient to purchase additional health insurance and will allow the patient to use monthly income to pay the bill. The patient pay amount to the nursing home will decrease accordingly. This provision allows the patient to make sure his or her needs are met. For example the patient may purchase vision or dental insurance. The nursing home will not provide the service but can arrange transportation to the provider.

The importance of complete coverage cannot be overstated. One dentist who specializes in dementia and nursing home patients, Dr. Katherine Martin, observed that over 25% of nursing home patients have serious dental needs. Even a three month stay without daily dental hygiene can cause a patient to go from having healthy teeth to having serious tooth decay.

Medicaid Tip: Uncovered Medical Expenses – Use the "Patient Pay Amount"

Others are concerned that they must give up certain treatment since the nursing home does not provide it or Medicaid does not cover it. A too little known fact is that Medicaid will allow the patient's monthly co-pay, called the "patient pay amount," to be used to pay for "non-covered service." Here is the word right from the Michigan Medicaid department's publication "Know Your Rights -- Your Medicaid Care And Coverage In A Nursing Facility":

• A doctor must document that the medical service is needed.

• Medicaid may limit the amount you can deduct from your patient-pay to obtain non-covered services.

• The provider of the service will bill you or the person handling your funds.

• It is up to you to pay the bill. Your monthly patient-pay amount is the most you will have to pay each month toward paying off a medical bill.

• You present a copy of the bill to your home. The bill will go towards your patient-pay amount for the next month. If the bill is less than your patient-pay amount, you must pay the rest of your patient-pay amount to the home.

• If you wish, you may payoff a bill that is more than your monthly patient-pay amount. This will result in lowering or replacing your monthly amount the following month(s). After you have received credit for the total bill you paid, your patient-pay amount will go back to the amount it was before you paid off the bill. See the example below. Example:

Your January patient-pay amount is: $200

You pay a medical bill of: $500

Your February patient-pay amount is: $0 because the paid bill will go against your February patient-pay amount of $200

Your March patient-pay amount is: $0

Your April patient-pay amount is: $100

Your May patient-pay amount is $200

You must give the nursing home a copy of the bill each month. In this example, February, March, and April.

There it is, from "the horse's mouth." Medicaid will cover all current medical needs.

Medicaid Tip: "Pre-eligibility Medical Expenses" – Use the "Patient Pay Amount"

Medical bills of the applicant incurred up to 90 days prior to the application for Medicaid may be paid out of the applicant's income. This is the result of a lawsuit the Michigan Elder Law attorneys supported. "Pre-Eligibility Medical Expenses" (PEME) are those that were incurred in the three months prior to application for Medicaid. The medical expense(s) must be:

- Unpaid, and an obligation still exists to pay.
- Cannot be from a month where Medicaid eligibility existed.
- Cannot be covered by a third party source (public or private).
- Cannot be from a month in which a divestment penalty has been imposed.
- Cannot have been used previously as a pre-eligibility medical expense to offset a patient pay amount.
- Can include cost of room and board for Medicaid long term care (LTC) facilities, remedial care and other medical expenses recognized by Michigan law but not covered under the Michigan state plan.

Special approval from the Medicaid Lansing office must obtained before the patient pay amount may be used to pay on these bills. You will need to work with the nursing home, your healthcare provider and your Medicaid worker.

So, you might use the spend down money for bills other than medical. Caution, though: this only works if the application is *approved*. Consult with an attorney.

Medicaid Rules for Married Couples
(Yes. You can save everything.)

Special rules apply to married couples due to the Spousal Impoverishment provisions of the Medicare Catastrophic Act. Where one spouse needs nursing home care and the other remains in the community, the law provides that the "community spouse" will be allowed enough savings to remain independent. The law recognizes that it makes little sense to impoverish both spouses when only one needs Medicaid assistance for nursing home care.

Assets, Excluded and Countable

Medicaid considers the assets, property and money, of both husband and wife. The couple gathers all of their countable assets together in a review. Excluded assets, discussed above, are not counted. The at-home or "community spouse" is allowed to keep *one-half of all countable assets.* In 2018 the *minimum is $24,720* and the *maximum is $123,600.* This allowance is called the <u>Community Spouse Resource Allowance</u> (CSRA). The remaining "half" of the countable assets must be "spent down" until $2,000 or less remains.

To make it clear let's look at two hypothetical couples, the Smiths and the Joneses. Medicaid requires them to disclose the amount of assets they had on the "snapshot date." That is the date the applicant, here the husband, began a stay of 30 days or longer in a hospital and or nursing home - in other words "long term care."

Let's assume that the Smiths had $100,000.00 in countable assets. The Joneses have $250,000.00. How much is the spend down and how much is at risk of being lost to long term care?

Smith		**Jones**	
Countable Assets on "Snapshot Date"	$100,000.00	Countable Assets on "Snapshot Date"	$250,000.00
Community Spouse Allowance (CSRA) *half of countable assets*	$50,000.00	Community Spouse Allowance (CSRA) *-maximum allowance*	$123,600.00
Nursing home spouse allowance	$2,000.00	Nursing home spouse allowance	$2,000.00
"Spend down"	$48,000.00	"Spend down"	$124,400.00

Comments. Note that the "spend down" does not mean how much they will spend. It refers to how much lower the countable assets must be before Medicaid will assist. The Smith's spend down is $48,000. Does that mean they only need to spend $48,000? No. They may actually spend much more.

Suppose the Smiths' total income is $2,800.00 per month. Mrs. Smith lives on just $800 per month and the remaining $2,000 goes to the nursing home. The average cost of nursing home care in Michigan in 2018 is $8,261 per month. That means she would have to take $6,261 out of savings every month. How long will it take for her to spend $48,000 of savings? In less than 8 months it would be gone. Her total expense would be over $64,000 since she would be spending income AND savings. It is possible for her to capture and save **all** of this money

Note that in the Jones case the community spouse is not "allowed" half of the countable assets. That would be $125,000. Instead her allowance is $123,600 because that is the *maximum* Community Spouse Resource Allowance (CSRA).

Must Mrs. Smith and Jones actually spend their savings? No. They could protect it by some examples we cover below. Note, there are additional ways to save money. See an experienced elder law attorney to learn what is available to you.

Income

Under Medicaid the nursing home resident's income goes to the nursing home. However Medicaid will first allow: $60 per month for personal needs; amount needed pay health insurance premiums; and the spousal allowance. The remainder is his "patient pay amount."

The Community Spouse Income Allowance (CSIA) "allows" the at-home spouse income from the patient according to a set schedule. The allowance considers how much income s/he has and adds patient income if needed. The minimum monthly income is $2,030 and the maximum is $3,090. The higher amount considers "excess shelter expense."

To illustrate, assume the at-home spouse receives $800 per month in Social Security and a small pension. Also assume that her monthly needs are calculated to be the minimum of $2,030. She is $1,230 short each month, as shown in the following chart:

$2,030.00   at-home spouse's minimum income allowance

($800.00)   at-home spouse's pension and Social Security

$1,230.00   Short fall

In this case, the community spouse will be allowed $1,230 (the shortfall amount) per month from her husband's income to meet the basic allowance of $2,030. She may be allowed more under an "excess shelter allowance." If the resident's income is higher than $1,230, the remainder (after his other deductions) would go to the nursing home as his patient pay amount. If it is less than $1,230 then she would only be allowed what he has in income and there would be no patient pay amount.

Where the spouse's income is less than the CSIA, Medicaid does not make up the difference in payment to the spouse.

The spouse may be allowed more of the resident's income by an "excess shelter expense allowance." This is triggered if the home expense (taxes, insurance and mortgage expense, or rent if the spouse is in an apartment) is more than Medicaid's standard allowance. Paying rent or mortgage usually triggers the excess shelter allowance so the spouse receives more of the resident's income and less goes to the nursing home.

Once again, there are other options the couple can pursue. Consider the following case studies[3]:

Case Study No. 1
Medicaid Planning for Married People

Ralph and Alice were high school sweethearts who lived in Livonia, Michigan their entire adult lives until they retired to Florida. Two weeks ago Ralph and Alice celebrated their 67th Anniversary. Alice has been struggling to care for Ralph, which is a round the clock job. He has Alzheimer's. Recently Alice heard some noise at 2:00 a.m. and got up to see Ralph out in the car and driving off. She called the police immediately. He was found a hours later. He was 20 miles from home and drove his car in a ditch. He got pretty banged up, they took him to the hospital and now he is in "rehab" at a nursing home. His Alzheimer's dementia got much worse. She will not be able to take him home unless he improves. The children want Alice to move back to Michigan and find a nursing home near them. She thinks she should, but she feels she has no alternative but to bring him back home. They cannot afford a nursing home!

Ralph and Alice were thrifty and always tried to save something each month. Their savings total $120,000, not including their house, are as follows:

Savings Account........	$35,000.00
CD's.	$65,000.00
Money Market Account.	$17,000.00
Checking Account.	$ 3,000.00
Residence -no mortgage.	$130,000.00

Ralph gets a Social Security check of $1260 each month. Ralph also gets a pension check of $650 a month. Alice's check is $680. Her eyes fill with tears as she says, "At $8,200 to the nursing home every month, our entire life savings will be gone in months!" What's more, she's afraid she won't be able

---

1. A Note about the Case Studies. No client information was used in the case studies. We do not publicize the confidential information of our clients. The studies are fictional examples of the application of Medicaid rules. You need not be concerned that your private information will be publicized in any way.

to pay her monthly bills, because a neighbor told her that the nursing home will be entitled to all of Ralph's Social Security check.

There is good news for Alice. It's possible she can keep everything – all of their assets and all of the income and still have the state Medicaid program pay Ralph's nursing home costs. The process is very complicated and she will need help.

To apply for Medicaid, she will have to go through the Department of Health and Human Services (DHS). If she does things strictly according to the way DHS tells her, she will only be able to keep about half of their assets, which is the "CSRA." Plus, they may only allow her community spouse income allowance, "CSIA", of $2,030 per month. She can do better.

Few people know that Medicaid has provisions for the spouse to keep all assets and income of husband and wife. A spouse may seek a court order directing the agency to allow such part of the assets and income. While the law allows the at home spouse to have it all, judges must be shown need for the resources. This requires the assistance of an experienced elder law attorney.

With proper advice and representation Alice will be able to avoid destitution and keep everything she and Ralph have worked so hard for. This is certainly an example of where knowledge of the rules, and how to apply them can be used to resolve a difficult dilemma.

Case Study No. 2
Spouse Returns Home With Veterans Benefits

Helen's husband Harold is 83 years old and a veteran of the Korean Conflict. Last month he suffered a paralyzing stroke and is now in post-hospital rehab. He is slowly improving and might be able to return to home but will need 24 hour assistance. An exhausted Helen seeks advice. Her hair is disheveled, dark circles have formed under her eyes. With her is daughter, assistant caregiver and all-around helper, Joan. She holds her mother's hand.

"The doctor says Harold needs long-term care in a nursing home," Helen says. "I can care for him in-home, if he doesn't have another stroke. Joan could help more but she is looking for work. I can pay for more help but I'm I afraid I will run out of savings. The social worker told me Harold should stay in the nursing home. I should just 'spend down.' I don't know what to do."

The good news is if Harold returns home that they can get help through the Veterans Administration. They may be able to get over $2,100 a month tax free and pay Joan for her help.

Before they go to the VA to inquire about "Aid and Attendance" they need to see an attorney experienced with the "special improved pension" program. If they make a claim prematurely they may be denied due to "excess net worth." The attorney will review their entire estate plan including financials and "estate planning" documents. The attorney can come up with a plan that will address their needs and qualify for the VA benefit.

Since Harold's condition is getting worse, it is possible that even with help he may have to go to a nursing home. That means they must have a plan that is flexible enough to provide immediate VA benefit, but yet not violate the Medicaid five year look back rules. They will not be able to use some strategies commonly used to gain VA benefits such as giving assets away or purchasing annuities.

There is another surprising problem that has to be addressed by the attorney: Medicaid considers paying children for helping out to be divestment of assets. For example, if she paid Joan $1,000 a month for 24 months, Medicaid would impose a "divestment penalty period" with the result that she would have to pay the nursing home care for almost three months before Medicaid would help. This problem can be completely avoided with a contract that meets Medicaid specifications.

Helen will be relieved. It can be done. She can bring Harold home. Joan can help and earn some money. VA will provide the benefit and there will be not problems with Medicaid should he need a nursing home within five years.

Single Elders
What of widowed or single persons in nursing homes? They have no spouse to act as patient advocate and protector. Children have their own families and jobs to attend to. But, what of the case where a child makes very large sacrifices to help her mother? The law allows her protection too.

Case Study No. 3
Planning for Veteran's Widow

Betty Johnson is exhausted. Four years ago her father died. She had been helping her parents for years, but since Dad died she has been the only support for her mother. At first, it was the daily little things: grocery shopping, laundry and cleaning, trips to the doctor, help with her medication, things like that. As her mom's health continued to deteriorate, Betty's burdens increased. Now her mother can no longer live alone.

Betty, a single mother, was laid-off from work. That means she has time to help her mother but she is running out of money. She is caught between her own needs, her family and her mother. None of her siblings can, or will, help. Betty fears she must place her mother in a nursing home so Betty can get a job. She has been looking for work but has had no offers. The last six months have been brutal.

Mom has about $50,000 and would like to give it to Betty rather than to a nursing home. Betty, quite rightly, fears that such a gift would make her mother ineligible for Medicaid assistance if her mother soon needed a nursing home. And, it could outrage her siblings.

Betty made some inquiries about Veterans Benefits - dad was a wartime vet. She was hoping mom would qualify for the surviving spouse aid and attendance benefit of $1,176 per month. But she found that mom has too much money and not enough "unreimbursed medical expense." In VA jargon she does not have enough "UME."

Betty is quite distraught. "Is there anything else I can do?"

Yes. Betty can be paid for her services and *if properly done*, her mother can get the full VA benefit and not worry about Medicaid "divestment." For example if mom moves into Betty's home, then mom can pay her fair market value rent. But what is that? An "assisted living" facility cost can exceed $6,000 per month. These payments can be recognized by the VA as Unreimbursed Medical Expense potentially triggering the maximum payment. But will the payments be considered "divestment" if mom needs to apply for Medicaid? This is a very difficult matter but it can be done.

They will need a formal contract that meets VA and Medicaid specifications before any payment is made and application for benefits made. Mom's need for the services must be documented by medical proof. The rent paid must be carefully determined to avoid a Medicaid finding of "divestment of assets." It can be done.

If Betty moves into Mom's home and provides enough care to keep Mom out of the nursing home, then Medicaid may allow mom to give Betty her home. However, they must do everything exactly right.

Note that "Medicaid planning" is not complete without family planning. To ensure family harmony, all family members should be involved in the process. It is plain that professional assistance will be needed *immediately*.

Disabled Children

There are a number of strategies that could be helpful. With any Medicaid planning it's especially important to seek the assistance of a knowledgeable Elder Law attorney to avoid violation of the Medicaid or tax rules. One can be assured that the plan selected will result in the greatest benefit for all without unintended consequences.

Sometimes planning must consider the family of the nursing home resident as well as the resident. For example, some children never gain independence – they remain forever dependent on their parents. What can be done in such a case?

Case Study No. 4
A Trust for a Disabled Child

For years Margaret and Sam took care of their daughter Sharon. She is disabled and receives SSI (Supplemental Security Income). Three years ago Sam died and their other daughter Beverly began helping Margaret and Sharon. Until he died Sam was Margaret's caregiver. She has Alzheimer's. That's when Beverly stepped up as her mother's agent under her durable power of attorney. Mom's health has deteriorated to the point that Beverly had to place her in a nursing home. Beverly is paying the nursing home $8,261 per month. Mom and Dad always wanted to leave something for Sharon. Now Beverly is worried that there will not be any money left for the care of Sharon.

Beverly is satisfied with the nursing home that Mom is in. The facility has a Medicaid bed available and Medicaid would pay the bill if she were eligible. However, according to the information Beverly got from the social worker, Mom is $48,000 away from Medicaid eligibility. She wishes there were a way to save the money for Sharon. There is.

If Margaret executed a comprehensive elder law power of attorney then Beverly can consult an Elder law attorney to set up a *"special needs trust"* with the $48,000 to provide for Elizabeth. As soon as she does Mom will be eligible for Medicaid, Elizabeth will not lose her SSI benefits and her future security will be assured.

Note that most powers of attorney do not allow transfer of assets to qualify for government benefits and the creation of a trust. These are essential powers. The best bet is to work with an experienced elder law attorney as soon as Alzheimer's is diagnosed.

Medicaid and Divestment of Assets

Many people ask "Can't I give away $14,000 a year?" friends told her to simply "hide the money" and give it to Joan.

The friends are giving bad, dangerous and incomplete advice. Giving away money and not disclosing on an application for government benefits is criminal fraud. Here are two points they should consider:

First, Helen and Joan have confused federal gift tax law with the issue of *asset transfers and **Medicaid eligibility**.* A "gift" to a child in this case is actually a transfer of assets and Medicaid has very specific rules about such and whether those are "divestment."

A final thought about gifting: remember, when it's given away, it's given away. Studies have shown that "windfall" money received by gift, prize or lawsuit settlement is often gone within three years. In other words, even when children promise that money will be available when needed, their own "emergencies" may make them spend the money.

"Will I Lose My Home?"

Many people who apply for Medicaid benefits to pay for nursing home costs ask this question. For many, the home constitutes most of their life savings. Often it is all the couple has to pass on to their children.

Under Medicaid, the home is an excluded asset, up to a maximum value, *on application.* The 2018 maximum is $572,000 in equity if the applicant has no spouse or disabled child living there. Note that the amount owed on a mortgage lessens the equity in the home. The exclusion ends on death. If there is no spouse or other protected person living in the home, then the home may be the subject of the "Medicaid estate recovery" program to seek recovery of all Medicaid payments.

A home *can* be lost on "estate recovery." Here's how it works. After the death of the Medicaid recipient and spouse if there is one, the state may demand repayment of benefits. Virtually any property owned by the Medicaid recipient and spouse may be subject to payback. Because the home is the single largest "excluded" asset that is not spent down, it is the main target of estate recovery. Michigan started going after homes in July 2011. That's the bad news. The good news is that you can avoid the state's claim if you avoid probate without creating "divestment."

Even if the home and other property should go to probate some or perhaps all can be saved. However, it is better to avoid the problem in the first place. Fortunately, there are ways to protect the home and other property that transfers upon death.

The solutions can range from re-titling, selling or gifting assets, converting them to income, to setting up contracts or trusts. Seek help from an experienced Elder Law attorney to help you in your planning.

Case Study No. 5
The $200,000 Mistake?

The complexity of the Medicaid rules and the frequent changes are a recipe for expensive missteps. People of ordinary means can be financially ruined by a misunderstanding of Medicaid eligibility rules. Spouses are especially vulnerable. In the prior case studies we have focused on estate planning options under the Medicaid rules. That is not the complete picture. Great care must be exercised in completing and submitting the Medicaid application.

Larry Smith is in the nursing home. His wife Patricia wanted to know how much she would have to spend before she could apply for help from Medicaid. She consulted a neighborhood lawyer who was not an Elder Law attorney.

The lawyer reviewed and listed her assets. He told her that she need not count her home or car, at this time. Then he made a list of their assets and told her which would have to be sold and spent on the nursing home.

Assets of Mr and Mrs. Smith on Entry into Nursing Home	
Excluded Assets (need not be spent)	
$125,000.00	Home in Dearborn Hts.
$6,000.00	2008 Ford Crown Victoria
$131,000.00	**Total Excluded Assets**
COUNTABLE ASSETS (To be spent down)	
$180,000.00	Cottage on Lake Huron: Mr and Mrs. Smith deeded the property to themselves and their two children and spouses in June 2009. They are all joint owners.
$93,500.00	CDs and savings at Big Bank. The accounts are joint between husband, wife and daughter (added last year).

$10,000.00	Loan to son, after he was laid off to avoid foreclosure on his home, made five years ago. The whole amount is still owing, clients have not made demand for payment.
$40,000.00	Book value, 2011 Conquerer 36 foot motor home
$323,500.00	TOTAL COUNTABLE ASSETS
($123,600.00)	Minus Community Spouse Resource Allowance
$199,900.00	**TOTAL to be spent down**

Upon completion of the list the lawyer explained that Medicaid allows only one homestead. So, the cottage would have to be sold. Mrs. Smith told him it had been listed for sale for three months, but no offers have been received. He said it is still an asset as is the motor home. They would have to be sold before Medicaid would be approved. She could keep the Ford. Finally she would have to collect from her son. The lawyer advised he would have to be sued in court if he did not pay.

In summary the lawyer said she would have to spend down her countable assets to $123,600, the maximum spouse allowance. She would have to spend $199,900! As we have seen before there are a number of ways to protect assets. But the unanswered question is "Did the lawyer make a mistake in his assessment?"

Did the lawyer make a mistake by counting the following assets?

$180,000.00   Cottage on Lake Huron

$10,000.00   Loan to son

$40,000.00   2011 Conquerer 36 foot motor home

$230,000.00   TOTAL

Maybe. He should have considered whether these were assets deemed "unavailable, non-salable or excluded." It is possible they should not be counted at all. If she consults an Elder Law attorney *she may not have to spend anything at all* on the nursing home. Mrs. Smith can choose among her options and decide how to best spend her own money and protect her family.

Conclusion

There are a number of strategies that applicants can use to qualify for Medicaid and still preserve some or all of their lifetime savings. The spouse and family can be protected.

These strategies are legal. They are moral. They are ethical.

Remember: the applicant *is a taxpayer*. It is impossible to have accumulated enough to require spend down without having paid taxes over a lifetime. It is only right that this taxpayer gets the benefits paid for by a lifetime of taxes.

You have the right to choose which options you will use and which you will not. This is akin to the millionaire visiting his tax advisor. Nobody would expect the tax advisor to say "You have saved enough. You should pay more taxes." The millionaire would expect the tax advisor to tell about all "deductions, credits and exemptions" that he could take and save money on taxes

Nobody should tell a family of modest means that they should not save their money. The family has every right to. Medicaid is like the tax code with "deductions, credits and exemptions." Please be advised, however, that Medicaid planning requires a great deal of knowledge of the current rules and practices of the system. They do change yearly and sometimes more often. Work with an experienced advisor who can advise you accurately.

Now, it's up to you

We hope we have met our goal of helping you to be an informed, powerful patient advocate. You will successfully get through the Medicare process, the discharge planning process and selecting a long term care facility, and finally, arranging payment without "going broke."

We wish you the best.

Long Term Care: Nursing Home, Or?

Whether your family member has gone through Medicare skilled care or you are considering that your patient can no longer live independently, you face a choice: assisted living or nursing home? Some folks recall the time when a person could not live at home they had to go to a nursing home. There was no other choice and that is why we call it a nursing *home*. Now there is a choice. There is a wide array of "assisted living facilities" that provide an alternative to the institutional care of a nursing home.

What Is the Difference Between Assisted Living and a Nursing Home?

First, you should know what a nursing home is and what it is not. Many families find very nice "memory care" or "dementia care" facilities that charge almost as much per month as a nursing home. These are generally known as "assisted living facilities." They seem to offer many services including on-premises home health services. Some present the question: "What about these assisted living facilities that I hear about? Are those new kinds of nursing homes?" The short answer is "No," but here is the more complete answer. What is the difference?

The first thing to understand is that an *assisted living facility* is not a medical treatment facility. Providers of medical services must be specifically licensed. While assisted living facilities may offer much in services, and may even have a nurse on duty during the day, they may not offer medical treatment. Since not all people need the 24 hour medical service that a nursing home offers, a brief review of each may be helpful.

Assisted Living

The term *assisted living* has a common sense meaning that a facility provides assistance to a resident in an apartment. This assistance may cover meals, housekeeping and laundry, more or less. A facility need not obtain a license to open and call itself "assisted living" though some do. In Michigan we have the following kinds of assisted living facilities:

Unlicensed. There are no regulations stating what the facility must do for its residents. This is the majority of assisted living facilities.

Licensed Adult Foster Care. Some facilities are licensed as Adult Foster Care Facilities. These may be certified for up to 20 people. Many are converted homes in single family neighborhoods and these are *limited to six residents*. The license of an adult foster home requires that each resident receive a written care agreement and that the facility follow a physician's health care plan. The facility is also required to promote independent living. The facility does not render medical treatment and cannot accept or retain a "patient" or person who requires continuous nursing care. That is the province of the nursing home.

Licensed Home for the Aged. This is a licensed facility with over 21 beds, that offers meals three times a day including therapeutic diets, laundry service, 24 hour staff, and assistance with personal care to persons over age 60. It, too, is required to promote independent living. The facility may not accept a resident with serious mental disturbance or one who needs intensive 24 hour nursing care.

State law provides residents of the above licensed facilities with a list of legal rights, the same as nursing home residents. A resident who feels that his/her rights have been violated or is not receiving proper care may file a complaint with either the Michigan Long Term Care Ombudsman or Department of Health and Human Services. See the *Resources* section in the back of this book.

Nursing Home

A *nursing home* is very different legally from an assisted living facility. It must be licensed before it can operate and it is extensively regulated by state and federal law in all aspects of the building and the delivery of care and medical treatment to the patients-residents. Most, but not all, nursing homes obtain certification to operate as "skilled nursing facility" and that means it has been certified to provide Medicare paid treatment for up to 100 days post-hospitalization. Most, but not all, are certified to receive payment for care for those residents who are in "Medicaid beds."

Regulation and care in a nursing home is complete. All of the following services are covered by regulation:
 (a) Admission, discharge, and transfer of patients;
 (b) Categories of patients accepted and not accepted by the home;
 (c) Clinical records;
 (d) Physician services;
 (e) Nursing services;
 (f) Dietary services;
 (g) Rehabilitative services;
 (h) Pharmaceutical services;
 (i) Diagnostic services;
 (j) Consultation services; (k) Dental services;
 (l) Podiatry services;
 (m) Social services, including counseling services;
 (n) Mental health services;
 (o) Diversional activities;
 (p) Interdisciplinary patient care planning;
 (q) Discharge planning;
 (r) Care of patients in an emergency, during a communicable disease episode, when critically ill, or when mentally disturbed.

The nursing home resident's rights are extensively protected even before admission. Federal and Michigan law regulate admission contracts for facilities that participate in Medicare and Medicaid. Once admitted, patients are protected by the Patients' Bill of Rights under Michigan law and the federal Nursing Home Reform Act of 1987. The nursing home is required to maintain the patient at the *"highest practicable level of functioning"* unless decline is medically unavoidable. In addition a "discharge" from a nursing home is strictly controlled by law and regulation. Residents have a long list of rights, *see below.*

How Do I Choose between Assisted Living and Nursing Home?
Sometimes you will have a choice between a nursing home and an assisted living facility. A nursing home can, by definition, offer "memory care" and "dementia care." How do you decide? Here's how you can make that decision.

If a person does not have extensive medical needs but cannot live independently then assisted living may offer a more residential option than a nursing home would. A person with advanced Alzheimer's Disease may be otherwise healthy but needs a safe place to live where needs can be met 24 hours a day. Some facilities specialize in care for Alzheimer's disease or other memory problems. Some are large facilities that offer much social stimulation and interaction. Others are much smaller and do not have the array of services but offer a more home-like setting. "Adult foster homes" may have only six residents and are often in residential neighborhoods. Finally, the monthly charge of an assisted living facility may be less than a nursing home, but the resident will have to move when he runs out of money. So, how does one choose?

At this time Medicaid will pay for a nursing home but not an assisted living facility, unless one is lucky enough to get a "Medicaid Waiver" slot through the "nursing facility transition program." That program pays part of the expense. Medicaid payment of the entire bill may seem a strong weight in favor of nursing home placement. The reality is that nursing home care is almost always institutional care whereas assisted living homes offer a more residential, apartment style of living. If it is truly a case of a choice then visit your local options.

Does a person really *need* nursing home level of care? Perhaps the best "objective" answer is to consult the "7 Doors Medicaid Screen" in the back of this book. It will tell you if the need is serious enough to qualify for nursing home payment by Medicaid. Medicaid will not pay for people who do not truly need a nursing home. If there is a question of whether the patient's condition can improve, you may have a doctor perform a geriatric assessment. This is a complete review of the person's medical condition, including medications and diet. Many elders' health can improve by making adjustments to their current regimen.

How to Select a Nursing Home

If your family member cannot live at home or assisted living any longer then the only choice is a nursing home. We can say that there are good and bad nursing homes. But, your conclusion will ultimately be based on your experience with a facility. A major part of that is the patient/resident's adaptation to the nursing home environment. The first factor then is the person you will be placing.

First: How Well Do You Know the Patient?
We often know little about those with whom we do not live. Perhaps you are helping an aunt or uncle, or just a friend. Even children may not know their parents as adults – they may still relate to them as "mom and dad." Children may live in different states and have not closely observed their parents in years since going off and starting their own home. Then, when crisis strikes they come back to find a frail elderly person about whom they know little of their every day life.

If you have not lived with your loved one, you may consider the following questions before or during placement. You will want to be ready to observe any changes that are due to a lack of good care. Here, we will use the feminine gender for ease of reference.

> With whom did your relative/friend live before coming to the nursing home?
> About how often have you seen her?
> Are you familiar with her preferences and daily routines when she was more
> independent and more able to make choices and express preferences?
> > Does she enjoy any particular activities or hobbies?
> > Does she tend to be more social or solitary?
> > What types of social and recreational activities does she prefer?
> > Did she work or volunteer in or out of the home?
> What are her:
> > Eating habits, food likes and dislikes?
> > Sleeping habits, alertness at different times of the day?
> > Religious/spiritual activities?
> > Things that give her pleasure?
> How would you describe the resident's lifelong general personality?
> > Is she thought to be quiet, happy, argumentative, etc.?
> > How did she generally adapted to change, prior to the current disability?
> > How, for example, did the resident react to moving to a new residence,
> > > to losing a loved one, and to other changing life situations?
> > Is she talkative or usually quiet, likely to express herself or not?

Two Ways to Choose a Nursing Home

Perhaps the quickest way to review a home is through www.Medicare.gov website in the "find a nursing home" section and choose one based on the rating. The second, and more traditional, is to simply choose one that is close by to family members who will visit the resident. The best is a combination of both.

Review Ratings on Medicare.gov

You may look up the nursing home on the federal government's Medicare web site, by using their "find nursing home" search:

http://www.medicare.gov/nursinghomecompare/search.html

You can select homes by zip code or city and state. You can review a summary report of the latest survey. You will find an interpretation of the rating, for example rating violations by number, pervasiveness and severity. Medicare has a star rating system on three criteria: staffing, health inspections and quality measures. A home may rate from one to five stars. You can use the star rating as a means to choose between two homes. In general a home should not be chosen on the basis of the number of stars. The first choice should be by proximity or ease of visitation. See the comments about "location" below.

Nursing Home Compare "Quality Measures"

The Medicare web site nursing home compare gives additional insight to the particular home by offering quality measures. It shows the percent of residents suffering from a number of conditions that the searcher may select. It allows the advocate to focus on a particular condition or see overall how the residents fare. The measures show how the facility compares, on the average, with other homes in the state. This can be due to the type of patient the nursing home has, for example more post-hospital rehabilitation than long term patients, or a "specialty" in treatment of difficult issues such as advanced bed sores. The advocate can use the quality measures in selection of a home and after selection of monitoring particular conditions.

Review the Latest State Survey

You will find that part of the Medicare star rating is based on the state annual survey of the home done by the State of Michigan Department of Consumer and Industry Services. You can ask to see a copy of that report. The home is supposed to have notice of it posted in a prominent place and available for review. How do you evaluate a home by reviewing the survey report? You may find it confusing and hard to interpret, *e.g.*, how serious is a deficiency? Once again, you will find the Medicare website helpful here. You can review the rating along with their assessment of how serious any violation is. You can also speak to the nursing home representative about steps they have taken to address the deficiencies reported.

Location

Sometimes the patient advocate finds that the only home with a vacancy that is convenient for visitation is lower in overall measures than others. The importance of active involvement in the care process including frequent visitation cannot be overstated. Most advocates would agree it is better to have a patient in a "poorer" home where frequent visitation is possible versus a "better" home that is so far away the patient can only be visited on weekends.

As a practical guide, choose a nursing home that you can visit on 10 minutes notice. That way you can run over there "at the drop of a hat." Good care requires constant monitoring. Daily visitation by a family member is almost mandatory. Your family member will not get good care if you visit only on the weekends. That is why being close is important. You want to be able to make a quick "pop in" visit to check up. You want to be able to get there immediately in case something bad happens. Remember even the best of nursing homes require oversight. There is no "set and forget."

Consider a hypothetical. Suppose you live in Rochester Hills, your brother lives in Plymouth and a sister lives in Royal Oak. Now the Lake Orion Nursing Center is a top rated facility but it would be very difficult for your brother or sister to get to. In the same way the Star Manor of Northville is top rated and would be convenient for your brother to get to, but is not for anybody else. You might try to find a nursing home that would be convenient for two of you. Marycrest Manor in Livonia may be doable for yo1ur brother and sister. Or, you might look at Woodward Hills in Bloomfield Hills, while not top rated and it has few Medicaid certified beds, it might be doable for you and your sister.

Visit the Home and Make Your Own Review the Homes

You will want to record your own impressions. You can use our Nursing Home Evaluation Checklist in the back of the book to make an informed record of your judgment. In addition to your own observations you should speak with family members who are visiting residents and ask about their experience with the home.

Select the Home

Once you are armed with your own findings, have spoken with residents, family and staff and reviewed the reports, you *will* be confident you have made the best possible choice.

Nursing Home Evaluation Checklists
Copyright Jim Schuster 2018

Record your observations as soon as possible, scoring your answers on a scale from Poor to Excellent or 1 to 5. Use the book as an original and make as copies as needed.

Name of Nursing Home: _____

Dates Visited Home: _____   Average Score :_____

The questions: Some may not lend themselves to scoring, an expected answer may be a simple yes or no. Score your impressions. Feel free to select those questions you wish to ask and to give more importance or weight to your particular areas of concern. Use the following guide for numbers: Poor = 1, Excellent = 5

A.   LOCATION

1   How convenient is the nursing home's location to   1 2 3 4 5
family members who *will* visit the resident ?

B. QUESTIONS FOR THE ADMISSIONS PERSON
After you have raised your questions with the admission person, test them by your observations or ask the same questions of residents and family members.

1   Are there rules in this facility? Do residents have   1 2 3 4 5
input?

2   Does the facility have a resident bed-time and a   1 2 3 4 5
wake-up time in the morning? Can residents choose
what time to go to bed and wake up?

3   Can residents have their own belongings here if they   1 2 3 4 5
choose to do so? What about their own furniture?

4   What is policy if personal belongings are missing?   1 2 3 4 5

5   Is mail delivery prompt? Does resident mail arrive   1 2 3 4 5
unopened?

6   What provision does the facility make to   1 2 3 4 5
accommodate the residents' legal rights such as
voting and making an advance directive and
appointing a patient advocate?

7	What effort does the facility make to assure privacy rights of residents?	1 2 3 4 5
8	Is there a secure area where a resident with Alzheimer's or other dementia can safely wander?	1 2 3 4 5
9	Is there a separate Alzheimer's or dementia care unit?	1 2 3 4 5
10	Does staff have training in various diseases of aging (Alzheimer's, Parkinson's etc.)? How often?	1 2 3 4 5
11	What is facility policy toward a staff member who is rude to residents?	1 2 3 4 5
12	Are residents involved in making decisions about nursing care, medical treatment and activities?	1 2 3 4 5
13	Do residents get permanent assignment of staff?	1 2 3 4 5
14	How good is the nursing home's record for employee retention?	1 2 3 4 5
15	What happens if a resident refuses care or treatment (such as a bath or certain medication)?	1 2 3 4 5
16	Do residents choose their own physician?	1 2 3 4 5
17	Does the facility accept Medicare and Medicaid?	1 2 3 4 5
18	Do residents have input into the selection of the activities offered?	1 2 3 4 5
19	Outside of the formal activity programs, are there opportunities for residents to socialize with other residents?	1 2 3 4 5
20	What method is used in selecting roommates?	1 2 3 4 5
21	Does the facility have an active family council?	1 2 3 4 5
22	Are *State Survey Results* readily available?	1 2 3 4 5
23	Have deficiencies reported in the state survey been corrected?	1 2 3 4 5

C. OBSERVATIONS AND QUESTIONS FOR RESIDENTS AND FAMILY

After you have spoken with the Admissions team, you will want to make your own observations. You will see if the reality matches their words and assurances.

1	Do corridors have handrails? Are handrails affixed to walls, intact, and free of splinters?	1 2 3 4 5
2	Is the facility free of objectionable odors and resident areas well ventilated?	1 2 3 4 5
3	Are nonsmoking areas smoke free? Are the smoking areas comfortable for residents who smoke?	1 2 3 4 5
4	Is it pest free and clean (walls, floors, drapes, furniture)?	1 2 3 4 5
5	Are housekeeping/hazards, compounds, and other chemicals stored to prevent resident access?	1 2 3 4 5
6	Is there a functioning call system in residents' bathing areas and toilet areas?	1 2 3 4 5
7	Is there room at and between tables for both residents and aides for those who need assistance with meals?	1 2 3 4 5
8	Are dining and activity rooms adequately furnished?	1 2 3 4 5
9	Are residents assisted with dining or with activities when necessary?	1 2 3 4 5
10	Is the resident equipment in common areas sanitary, orderly, and in good repair?	1 2 3 4 5
11	Are adequate accommodations made for resident privacy, during medical treatment and visiting with family?	1 2 3 4 5
12	Are rooms safe and comfortable in the following areas: Room temperature, water temperature, sound level, and lighting?	1 2 3 4 5
13	Are bedding, bath linens and closet space adequate for resident needs?	1 2 3 4 5

14   Is environment homelike, comfortable and attractive? Are accommodations are made for resident personal items and modifications?   1 2 3 4 5

15   Are residents with physical limitations (e.g. walker, wheel-chair) able to move around their rooms?   1 2 3 4 5

16   Do residents appear well groomed and reasonably attractive (e.g. clean clothes, neat hair, free from facial hair)?   1 2 3 4 5

17   Does staff treat residents respectfully and listen to resident requests?   1 2 3 4 5

18   Is staff is responsive to resident requests and call bells?   1 2 3 4 5

19   While staff are giving care, do they include resident in conversation or do staff talk to each as if resident is not there?   1 2 3 4 5

20   Is the Administration responsive to the Family Council?   1 2 3 4 5

21   Is information about Medicare, Medicaid and contacting advocacy agencies posted?   1 2 3 4 5

D. Comments / Observations / Persons Spoken With

_____

_____

_____

_____

Nursing Homes in Southeast Michigan

In the previous pages, we've talked about how to find the right nursing home, how to get good care there, and how to pay for it without going broke. But where do you actually start looking? Where should you begin your search?

To assist you, we've compiled a list of the nursing homes in Southeast Michigan arranged by county. The listings contain the name and address of the facility along with the telephone number. We have also included information on whether the facility accepts Medicare and Medicaid.

For more information on a particular nursing home visit Medicare web site and review the "compare nursing homes" information: www.medicare.gov/nhcompare/

Pay close attention to the "star rating" of a nursing home. See our "How to Select a Nursing Home" section earlier in the book.

The information in the following listing is current as of February 2018. All attempts have been made to assure accuracy. If you spot any error, please contact the publisher, Jim Schuster, at the address on the inside cover.

How to Read the Tables

Most of the information is straightforward but many people question what does "**Medicare Only**" etc., mean? Those column notations refer to the "certification" of certain beds. Medicare or Medicaid will only pay for care rendered in those identified beds. Of course, you can still use your own money and "private pay" for care in those beds. The "**Licensed Only**" column identifies beds that have no additional certification and hence we refer to those as private pay beds.

Note: Homes in Macomb, Oakland and Wayne Counties are listed first. Homes in Lapeer, Livingston, Monroe, St. Clair and Washtenaw follow.

— Tri-county Nursing Homes —

MACOMB COUNTY Medicare or Medicaid refers to the beds certified for payment by each program	Total Beds	Medicare Only	Medicare and Medicaid	Medicaid Only	Licensed Only
ADVANTAGE LIVING CENTER - 22600 Armada Ridge Rd Armada, MI 48005 (586) 784-5322	67		67		
ADVANTAGE LIVING CENTER - 25375 Kelly Rd. Roseville, MI 48066 (586) 773-6022	169		169		
ADVANTAGE LIVING CENTER 12250 E. 12 Mile Rd. Warren, MI 48093 (586) 751-6200	144		144		
AUTUMN WOODS 29800 Hoover Rd. Warren, MI 48093 (586) 574-3444	293	17	276		
CHERRYWOOD NURSING & LIVING 34643 Ketsin Drive Sterling Heights, MI 48310 (586) 978-2280	180		180		
CHURCH OF CHRIST CARE CENTER 23575 15 Mile Rd. Clinton Township, MI 48035 (586) 791-2470	129		129		
CLINTON-AIRE HEALTHCARE CTR 17001 17 Mile Rd. Clinton Township, MI 48038 (586) 286-7100	132		127		5
EVANGELICAL HOME 14900 Shoreline Dr. Sterling Heights, MI 48313-2251 (586) 247-4700	112		112		
FATHER MURRAY NURSING CENTER 8444 Engleman Rd. Centerline, MI 48015 (586) 755-2400	231		231		
HEARTLAND HEALTHCARE CENTER - 38200 Schoenherr Rd. Sterling Heights, MI 48312 586-274-9044	163	137	26		
LAKEPOINTE CARE & REHAB CTR 37700 Harper Ave. Clinton Township, MI 48036 (586) 468-0827	134		134		

MACOMB COUNTY Medicare or Medicaid refers to the beds certified for payment by each program	Total Beds	Medicare Only	Medicare and Medicaid	Medicaid Only	Licensed Only
LAKESIDE MANOR 13990 Lakeside Circle, Sterling Heights, MI 48313 (586) 488-1400	66		66		
MARTHA T. BERRY CARE FACILITY 43533 Elizabeth Rd. Mt. Clemens, MI 48043 (586) 469-5265	217		217		
MEDILODGE OF RICHMOND 34901 Division Rd. Richmond, MI 48062 (586) 727-7562	126	12	114		
MEDILODGE OF STERLING HEIGHTS 14151 E. 15 Mile Rd. Sterling Heights, MI 48312 (586) 939-0200	295		295		
ORCHARD GROVE HEALTH CAMPUS 71150 Orchard Crossing Lane, Romeo, MI 48065 (586) 336-0102	55		55		
REGENCY AT SHELBY TOWNSHIP 7401 22 Mile Road Shelby Township, MI 48317 (586) 580-5500	116		116		
REGENCY MANOR NURSING CENTER 7700 McClellan UTICA, MI 48317 (586) 739-7700	39		39		
SANCTUARY AT FRASER VILLA 33300 Utica Rd. Fraser, MI 48026 (586) 293-3300	154	48	106		
SHELBY CROSSING HEALTH CAMPUS 13794 21 Mile Rd. Shelby Twp., MI 48315 586-532-2100	114		57		57
SHELBY NURSING CENTER 46100 Schoenherr Rd. Shelby Township, MI 48315 (586) 566-1100	212	168	44		
SHOREPOINTE NURSING CENTER 26001 E. Jefferson Avenue St. Clair Shores, MI 48081 (586) 779-7000	200	100	100		

MACOMB COUNTY Medicare or Medicaid refers to the beds certified for payment by each program	Total Beds	Medicare Only	Medicare and Medicaid	Medicaid Only	Licensed Only
ST. ANTHONY HEALTHCARE CENTER 31830 Ryan Rd. Warren, MI 48092 (586) 977-6700	142		142		
ST. MARY'S NURSING CTR 22601 E. Nine Mile Rd. St. Clair Shores, MI 48080 (586) 772-4300	101		101		
THE VILLA AT CITY CENTER 11700 E Ten Mile Rd Warren, MI 48089 (586) 759-5960	152		152		
THE VILLAGE OF EAST HARBOR 33875 Kiely Drive Chesterfield, MI 48047 (586) 725-6030	90	18	72		
WARREN WOODS REHAB. CTR 11525 E. 10 Mile Rd. Warren, MI 48089 (586) 759-0700	178		178		
WELLBRIDGE OF ROMEO, LLC 375 South Main Street Romeo, MI 48065 (586) 589-3800	124		124		
WINDEMERE PARK CENTER 31800 Van Dyke Avenue, Warren, MI 4809 (586) 563-1500	92		92		

OAKLAND COUNTY Medicare or Medicaid refers to the beds certified for payment by each program	Total Beds	Medicare Only	Medicare and Medicaid	Medicaid Only	Licensed Only
BELLBROOK 873 W. Avon Rd. Rochester Hills, MI 48307 (248) 656-3239	66	12	54		
BLOOMFIELD ORCHARD VILLA 7277 Richardson Rd. West Bloomfield, MI 48323 (248) 360-4443	50		50		
BOTSFORD CONT. HEALTH CTR. 21450 Archwood Circle Farmington, MI 48336-4702 (248) 477-7400	179	59	120		

OAKLAND COUNTY Medicare or Medicaid refers to the beds certified for payment by each program	Total Beds	Medicare Only	Medicare and Medicaid	Medicaid Only	Licensed Only
BOULEVARD HEALTH CENTER 3500 W. South Blvd. Rochester Hills, MI 48309 (248) 852-7800	186		186		
CAMBRIDGE EAST HEALTHCARE 31155 Dequindre Rd. Madison Heights, MI 48071 (248) 585-7010	154		154		
CAMBRIDGE NORTH HEALTHCARE 535 N. Main St. Clawson, MI 48017 (248) 435-5200	120		120		
CAMBRIDGE SOUTH HEALTHCARE 18200 W. 13 Mile Rd. Beverly Hills, MI 48025 (248) 647-6500	96		96		
CANTERBURY ON THE LAKE 5601 Hatchery Rd. Waterford, MI 48329 (248) 674-9292	128	48	80		
CATHERINE'S PLACE 28750 Eleven Mile Rd. Farmington Hills, MI 48336 (248) 473-7190	27		27		
CEDARBROOK BLOOMFIELD HILLS 41150 Woodward Avenue, Bloomfield Hills, MI 48304 (248) 955-4956					20
CLARKSTON SPECIALTY HEALTH 4800 Clintonville Rd. Clarkston, MI 48346 (248) 674-0903	120	28	92		
EVERGREEN HEALTH AND LIVING 19933 W. 13 Mile Rd. Southfield, MI 48076 (248) 203-9000	151	110	41		
FOX RUN VILLAGE 41215 Thirteen Mile Road Novi, Mi 48377 (248) 668-8720	88	38	6		44
GREENFIELD REHAB & NURSING 3030 Greenfield Rd. Royal Oak, MI 48073 (248) 288-6610	126		126		

OAKLAND COUNTY Medicare or Medicaid refers to the beds certified for payment by each program	Total Beds	Medicare Only	Medicare and Medicaid	Medicaid Only	Licensed Only
HEARTLAND HCC - BLOOMFIELD 2975 N. Adams Rd. Bloomfield Hills, MI 48304 (248) 645-2900	159	159			
HEARTLAND HCC OAKLAND 925 W. South Blvd TROY, MI 48085 (248) 729-4400	160	160			
HEARTLAND HCC W. BLOOMFIELD 6950 Farmington Rd. West Bloomfield, MI 48322 (248)661-1700	140	116	24		
LAHSER HILLS CARE CENTRE 25300 Lahser Rd. Southfield, MI 48034 (248) 354-3222	143		143		
LAKE ORION NURSING CENTER 585 E. Flint St. Lake Orion, MI 48362 (248) 693-0505	120		120		
LAKELAND CENTER 26900 Franklin Rd. Southfield, MI 48034 (248) 350-8070	91	38	53		
LOURDES NURSING HOME 2300 Watkins Lake Rd. Waterford, MI 48328 (248) 674-2241	108		108		
MAPLE MANOR REHAB CTR NOVI 31215 Novi Rd. Novi, MI 48377 (248)624-8800	72	72	72		
MARVIN & BETTY DANTO FAMILY HEALTHCARE CENTER 6800 W. Maple Rd. West Bloomfield, MI 48322 (248) 788-5300	155	50	105		
MEDILODGE OF FARMINGTON 34225 Grand River Ave. Farmington, MI 48335 (248) 477-7373	124	6	118		
MEDILODGE OF MILFORD 555 Highland Ave. Milford, MI 48381 (248)685-1460	111		111		

OAKLAND COUNTY Medicare or Medicaid refers to the beds certified for payment by each program	Total Beds	Medicare Only	Medicare and Medicaid	Medicaid Only	Licensed Only
MEDILODGE OF ROCHESTER HILLS. 1480 Walton Blvd. Rochester, MI 48309 (248) 651-4422	126	14	112		
MEDILODGE OF SOUTHFIELD 26715 Greenfield Rd. Southfield, MI 48076 (248) 557-0050	191		191		
MISSION POINT NURSING – HOLLY 313 Sherwood St, Holly, MI 48442	66		66		
NOTTING HILL OF W. BLOOMFIELD 6535 Drake Rd. W. Bloomfield, MI 48322 248-592-2000	120		120		
NOVI LAKES HEALTH CAMPUS 41795 W 12 Mile Road Novi, MI 48377	54		54		
OAKLAND MANOR NURSING CTR. 50 N Perry St, 1st Floor PONTIAC, MI 48342 (248) 221-5300	39	10			29
OAKLAND NURSING CENTER 22401 Foster Winter Drive Southfield Mi, 48075 (248) 423-5100	26		26		
OAKRIDGE MANOR NURSING CTR 3161 Hilton Rd. Ferndale, MI 48220 (248)547-6227	64	19	45		
REGENCY AT WATERFORD 1901 N. Telegraph Rd Waterford, MI 48328 (248)836-1000	150		150		
SOUTH LYON SENIOR CARE REHAB 700 Reynold Sweet Parkway South Lyon, MI 48178 (248)437-2048	74		74		
ST. ANNES MEAD 16106 West 12 Mile Road Southfield, MI 48076	29				29
THE MANOR, FARMINGTON HILLS 21017 Middlebelt Rd. Farmington Hills, MI 48336 (248) 476-8300	114		102		12

| OAKLAND COUNTY
Medicare or Medicaid refers to the beds certified for payment by each program	Total Beds	Medicare Only	Medicare and Medicaid	Medicaid Only	Licensed Only
THE MANOR OF NOVI 24500 Meadowbrook Rd. Novi, MI 48375 (248) 477-2000	140		140		
THE NEIGHBORHOODS WHITE LAKE 10770 Elizabeth Lake Road White Lake, MI 48386 (248) 618-4100	92		92		
THE VILLA AT GREEN LAKE 6470 Alden Dr Orchard Lake, MI 48324 (248) 363-4121	85		85		
THE VILLA – SILVERBELL ESTATES 1255 W SILVERBELL RD ORION, MI 48359 (248) 391-0900	106	12	94		
WELLBRIDGE OF NOVI, LLC 48300 11 Mile Road Novi, MI 48374 (248) 662-2300	100		100		
WELLBRIDGE OF ROCHESTER HILLS 252 Meadowfield Drive Rochester Hills, MI 48307 (248) 218-4800	100		100		
WEST BLOOMFIELD NURSING & CONVALESCENT CENTER 6445 W. Maple Rd. West Bloomfield, MI 48322 (248) 661-1600	172	89	83		
WEST HICKORY HAVEN 3310 W. Commerce Rd. Milford, MI 48380 (248) 685-1400	101		101		
WESTLAKE HEALTH CAMPUS 10765 Bogie Lake Rd. Commerce, MI 48382 (248) 363-9400	64		64		
WHITEHALL HEALTHCARE - NOVI 43455 W. 10 Mile Rd. Novi, MI 48375-3100 (248) 349-2200	82		82		
WOODWARD HILLS NURSING CTR 39312 Woodward Ave. Bloomfield Hills, MI 48304 (248) 644-5522	190	128	62		

WAYNE COUNTY Medicare or Medicaid refers to the beds certified for payment by each program	Total Beds	Medicare Only	Medicare and Medicaid	Medicaid Only	Licensed Only
ABERDEEN REHAB. NURSING CTR 5500 Fort Trenton, MI 48183 (734) 671-3500	198	20	105		73
ADVANTAGE LIVING CENTER 19840 Harper Ave. Harper Woods, MI 48225 (313) 881-9556	151		151		
ADVANTAGE LIVING CTR- Northwest 16181 Hubbell Ave. Detroit, MI 48235 (313) 273-8764	154	14	140		
ADVANTAGE LIVING CTR-REDFORD 25330 W. Six Mile Road Redford, MI 48240 (313) 531-6874	88	18	70	***	
ADVANTAGE LIVING - SAMARITAN 5555 Conner Avenue, Suite 4000 Detroit, Mi 48213 (313) 344-4100	120		120		
ADVANTAGE LIVING CTR - Southgate 15400 Trenton Rd. Southgate, MI 48195 (734) 284-4620	100		100		
ADVANTAGE LIVING CTR - WAYNE 4427 Venoy Rd Wayne, MI 48184 (734) 729-4436	179	32	147		
ALPHA MANOR NURSING HOME 440 E. Grand Blvd. Detroit, MI 48207 (313) 579-2900	80		80		
AMBASSADOR NURSING REHAB 8045 E. Jefferson Ave. Detroit, MI 48214 (313) 821-3525	176		176		
ANGELA HOSPICE CARE CENTER 14100 Newburgh Road Livonia, MI 4815	12				12
APPLEWOOD NURSING CENTER, 18500 Van Horn Rd. Woodhaven, MI 48183 (734) 676-7575	150		150		

WAYNE COUNTY Medicare or Medicaid refers to the beds certified for payment by each program	Total Beds	Medicare Only	Medicare and Medicaid	Medicaid Only	Licensed Only
AUTUMNWOOD OF LIVONIA 14900 Middlebelt Livonia, MI 48154 (734) 425-4200	142		142		
BEACONSHIRE NURSING CENTRE 21630 Hessel Rd. Detroit, MI 48219 (313) 534-8400	99	8	91		
BEAUMONT - OAKWOOD COMMON 16391 Rotunda Dr. Dearborn, MI 48120 (313) 253-9700	200	142	58		
BELLE FOUNTAIN NURSING REHAB. 18591 Quarry Rd. Riverview, MI 48192 (734) 282-2100	91		91		
BOULEVARD MANOR 464 E. Grand Blvd. Detroit, MI 48207 (313) 579-2255	87	19	68		
BOULEVARD TEMPLE 2567 W. Grand Blvd. Detroit, MI 48208 (313) 895-5340	124	54	70		
CAMELOT HALL CONVALESCENT 35100 Ann Arbor Trail Livonia, MI 48150 (734) 522-1444	142		122		20
EASTWOOD CONVALESCENT CTR 626 E. Grand Blvd. Detroit, MI 48207 (313) 923-5816	72		72		
FAIRLANE CARE REHAB CTR 15750 Joy Rd. Detroit, MI 48228 (313) 273-6850	205		205		
FOUR CHAPLAINS NURSING CARE 28349 Joy Rd. Westland, MI 48185 (734) 261-9500	103		103		
FOUR SEASONS NURSING CENTER 8365 Newburgh Rd. Westland, MI 48185 (734) 416-2000	180	20	160		

WAYNE COUNTY Medicare or Medicaid refers to the beds certified for payment by each program	Total Beds	Medicare Only	Medicare and Medicaid	Medicaid Only	Licensed Only
HAMILTON NURSING HOME 590 E. Grand Blvd. Detroit, MI 48207 (313) 921-1580	118		64		
HARTFORD NURSING REHAB. CTR 6700 W. Outer Dr. Detroit, MI 48235 (313) 836-1700	140	20	120		
HEARTLAND HCC-ALLEN PARK 9150 Allen Rd. Allen Park, MI 48101 (313) 386-2150	163	92	71		
HEARTLAND HCC-CANTON 7025 Lilley Road Canton, MI 48187 (734) 394-3100	150	126	24		
HEARTLAND HCC-DEARBORN HTS 26001 Ford Rd. Dearborn Heights, MI 48127 (313) 274-4600	124	92	32		
HEARTLAND HCC-GROSSE POINTE 21401 Mack Ave. Grosse Pointe, MI 48236 (586) 778-0800	80	71	9		
HEARTLAND HCC-LIVONIA - NE 29270 Morlock Livonia, MI 48152 (248) 476-0555	110	45	65		
HEARTLAND HCC-LIVONIA 28550 Five Mile Rd. Livonia, MI 48154 (734) 427-8270	142		142		
HEARTLAND HCC-PLYMOUTH 105 Haggerty Plymouth, MI 48170 (734) 455-0510	101	56	55		
HENRY FORD VILLAGE, INC. 15101 Ford Rd. Dearborn, MI 48126 (313) 582-2097	89	62	27		
HERITAGE MANOR NURSING CTR 9500 GRAND RIVER AVE DETROIT, MI 48204 (313) 491-7920	122	26	96		

WAYNE COUNTY Medicare or Medicaid refers to the beds certified for payment by each program	Total Beds	Medicare Only	Medicare and Medicaid	Medicaid Only	Licensed Only
HOPE HEALTHCARE CENTER 38410 Cherry Hill Rd. Westland, MI 48185 (734) 326-1200	129		129		
IMPERIAL HEALTH CARE CENTRE 26505 Powers Ave. Dearborn Heights, MI 48125 (313) 291-6200	265		265		
LAW-DEN NURSING HOME 1640 Webb Rd. Detroit, MI 48206 (313) 867-1719	100		100		
LIVONIA WOODS NURSING 33600 Luther Lane Livonia, MI 48154 (734) 421-6564	72		72		
MAPLE MANOR REHAB. CTR. 3999 Venoy Wayne, MI 48184 (734) 727-0440	59	47	12		
MARYCREST MANOR 15475 Middlebelt Rd. Livonia, MI 48154 (734) 427-9175	98		98		
MARYWOOD NURSING CARE CTR 36975 W. Five Mile Livonia, MI 48154 (734) 464-0600	103	79	24		
MEDILODGE OF PLYMOUTH, INC. 395 W. Ann Arbor Trail Plymouth, MI 48170 (734) 453-3983	39		39		
MEDILODGE OF TAYLOR, INC. 23600 Northline Rd. Taylor, MI 48180 (734) 287-8580	142	8	132		
OAKPOINTE CARE & REHAB. CTR 18901 Meyers Rd. Detroit, MI 48235 (313) 864-8481	133		133		
OMNI CONTINUING CARE 5201 Conner Rd. Detroit, MI 48213 (313) 571-5555	136		136		

WAYNE COUNTY Medicare or Medicaid refers to the beds certified for payment by each program	Total Beds	Medicare Only	Medicare and Medicaid	Medicaid Only	Licensed Only
PARKEAST HEALTHCARE CENTER 6232 Cadieux Rd. Detroit, MI 48224 (313) 886-2500	78	6	72		
QUALICARE NURSING HOME 695 E. Grand Blvd. Detroit, MI 48207 (313) 925-6655	96		96		
REGENCY AT CANTON 45900 Geddes Road Canton, MI 48188 (734) 707-6024	113		113		
REGENCY HEALTHCARE CENTRE 12575 S. Telegraph Rd. Taylor, MI 48180 (734) 287-4710	244		244		
REGENCY HEIGHTS-DETROIT 19100 West Seven Mile Rd. Detroit, MI 48219 (13) 533-5002	194		168		26
RIVERGATE HEALTH CARE CENTER 14041 Pennsylvania Ave. Riverview, MI 48193 (734) 284-7200	223		223		
RIVERGATE TERRACE 14141 Pennsylvania Ave. Riverview, MI 48193 (734) 284-8000	288		288		
RIVERVIEW HEALTH & REHAB 7733 E Jefferson Detroit, MI 48214 (313) 563-1500	176		176		
RIVERVIEW HEALTH REHAB NORTH 18300 E. Warren Ave. Detroit, MI 48224 (313) 343-8000	180		180		
SHEFFIELD MANOR NURSING CTR 15311 Schaefer Rd. Detroit, MI 48227 (313) 835-4775	106		106		
ST. FRANCIS NURSING CENTER 1533 Cadillac Detroit, MI 48214 313-823-0435	81		81		

WAYNE COUNTY Medicare or Medicaid refers to the beds certified for payment by each program	Total Beds	Medicare Only	Medicare and Medicaid	Medicaid Only	Licensed Only
ST. JAMES NURSING CENTER 15063 Gratiot Ave. Detroit, MI 48205 (313) 372-4065	143		143		
ST. JOSEPH'S HEALTHCARE CTR 9400 Conant Ave. Hamtramck, MI 48212 (313) 874-4500	169		169		
ST. JUDE NURSING CENTER 34350 Ann Arbor Trail Livonia, MI 48150 (734) 261-4800	64		64		
STAR MANOR OF NORTHVILLE 520 W. Main St. – P.O. BOX 206 Northville, MI 48167 (248) 349- 4290	37			37	
THE BAY AT CRANBROOK 5000 E. Seven Mile Rd. Detroit, MI 48234 (313) 366-2900	66		66		
THE BAY AT ELMWOOD 1881 E. Grand Blvd. Detroit, MI 48211 (313) 922-1600	120		120		
THE BAY AT WOODWARD 9146 Woodward Ave. Detroit, MI 48202 (313) 875-1263	110		110		
THE LODGE AT TAYLOR. 22950 Northline Rd. Taylor, MI 48180 (734) 287-1230	150		150		
THE RIVERS OF GROSSE POINTE 900 Cook Road Grosse Pointe Woods, MI 48236 (313) 821-7095	86		86		
THE VILLA - GREAT LAKES CROSSING 22811 W. Seven Mile Rd. Detroit, MI 48219 (313) 534-1440	98		98		
THE VILLA AT THE PARK 111 Ford Ave. Highland Park, MI 48203 (313) 883-3585	114		114		

WAYNE COUNTY Medicare or Medicaid refers to the beds certified for payment by each program	Total Beds	Medicare Only	Medicare and Medicaid	Medicaid Only	Licensed Only
TRANSITIONAL HEALTH OF WAYNE 34330 Van Born Rd. Wayne, MI 48184 (734) 721-0740	49	8	41		
WELLSPRING LUTHERAN SERVICE 28910 Plymouth Road Livonia, MI 48150 (734) 425-4814	88		88		
WEST OAKS CARE & REHAB CTR 22355 W Eight Mile Rd. Detroit, MI 48219 (313) 255-6450	102		102		
WESTLAND CONVALESCENT 36137 Warren Ave. Westland, MI 48185 (734) 728-6100	230		230		
WESTWOOD NURSING CENTER 16588 Schaefer Rd. Detroit, MI 48235 (313) 345-5000	112	9	99		13
WOODHAVEN RETIREMENT COMMUNITY 29667 Wentworth Livonia, MI 48154 (734) 261-9000	32	16	16		

— Nursing Homes Outside Metro-Detroit Area —

LIVINGSTON COUNTY Medicare or Medicaid refers to the beds certified for payment by each program	Total Beds	Medicare Only	Medicare and Medicaid	Medicaid Only	Licensed Only
CARETEL INNS OF BRIGHTON 1014 E. Grand River Brighton, MI 48116 (810) 220-5222	60	54	6		
MEDILODGE OF HOWELL 1333 W. Grand River Howell, MI 48843 (517) 548-1900	219		203		
MEDILODGE OF LIVINGSTON 3003 W. Grand River Howell, MI 48843 (517) 546-4210	139	22	117		
THE WILLOWS AT HOWELL 1500 Byron Road Howell, MI 48855 (517) 552-9323	56		56		
WELLBRIDGE OF BRIGHTON 2200 Dorr Rd. Howell, MI 48843 (517) 947-4400	88		88		
WELLBRIDGE OF PINCKNEY 664 South Howell Street, Pinckney, MI 48169 (734) 954-6700	100		100		

MONROE COUNTY Medicare or Medicaid refers to the beds certified for payment by each program	Total Beds	Medicare Only	Medicare and Medicaid	Medicaid Only	Licensed Only
FOUNTAIN VIEW OF MONROE 1971 N Monroe Street Monroe, MI 48162 (734) 243-8800	119		119		
HICKORY RIDGE OF TEMPERANCE 951 Hickory Creek Boulevard Temperance, MI 48182 (734) 206-8200	74		74		
IHM Senior Community (religious) 610 West Elm Avenue Monroe, MI 48162 (734) 241-3660	58		58		

MONROE COUNTY Medicare or Medicaid refers to the beds certified for payment by each program	Total Beds	Medicare Only	Medicare and Medicaid	Medicaid Only	Licensed Only
MAGNUMCARE OF MONROE 1215 N Telegraph Rd Monroe, MI 88162 (734) 242-4848	152	12	119		32
MEDILODGE OF MONROE, L L C 481 Village Green Lane Monroe, MI 48162 (734) 242-6282	103		103		
PROMEDICA MONROE SKILLED 700 Stewart Rd Monroe, MI 48161 (734) 240-1740	89		89		
WELLSPRING LUTHERAN NURSING 1236 S Monroe St Monroe, MI 48161 (734) 241-9533	122		122		

ST. CLAIR COUNTY Medicare or Medicaid refers to the beds certified for payment by each program	Total Beds	Medicare Only	Medicare and Medicaid	Medicaid Only	Licensed Only
MARWOOD MANOR NURSING HOME 1300 Beard St. Port Huron, MI 48060 (810) 982-9500	240		240		
MEDILODGE OF PORT HURON, INC. 5635 Lakeshore Fort Gratiot, MI 48059 (810) 385-7447	127	12	115		
MEDILODGE OF ST. CLAIR, INC. 4220 S. Hospital Drive East China, MI 48054 (810) 329-4736	172	45	127		
MEDILODGE OF YALE, INC. 90 Jean St. Yale, MI 48097 (810) 387-3226	115	12	103		
REGENCY ON THE LAKE - FT. GRATIOT 5669 Lakeshore Fort Gratiot, MI 48059 (810) 385-7260	174	44	130		

WASHTENAW COUNTY Medicare or Medicaid refers to the beds certified for payment by each program	Total Beds	Medicare Only	Medicare and Medicaid	Medicaid Only	Licensed Only
ARBOR HOSPICE (Residence) 2366 Oak Valley Drive, Ann Arbor, MI 48103					30
CARE GLACIER HILLS, 19 1200 Earhart Rd. Ann Arbor, MI 48105 (734) 769-0177	161	82	79		
CHELSEA RETIREMENT COMMUNITY 805 W. Middle St. Chelsea, MI 48118 (734) 475-8633	85	40	45		
EVANGELICAL HOME - SALINE 440 W. Russell Saline, MI 48176 (734) 429-9401	215		215		
GILBERT RESIDENCE 203 S. Huron St. Ypsilanti, MI 48197 (734) 482-9498	32			32	
HEARTLAND HCC-ANN ARBOR 4701 E. Huron River Drive Ann Arbor, MI 48105 (734) 975-2600	180	100	80		
REGENCY AT BLUFFS PARK 355 Huron View Blvd. Ann Arbor, MI 48103 734-887-8700	71		71		
REGENCY AT WHITMORE LAKE 8633 N. Main St. Whitmore Lake, MI 48189 (734) 449-4431	135		135		
SUPERIOR WOODS 8380 Geddes Road Ypsilanti, MI 48198 (734) 547-7600	94		94		
THE VILLA AT PARKRIDGE 28 S. Prospect St. Ypsilanti, MI 48198 (734) 483-2220	144		144		
WHITEHALL CTR OF ANN ARBOR 3370 Morgan Rd. Ann Arbor, MI 48108 (734) 971-3230	102	19	83		

– Resources –

Medicare Reviews of Discharge from Hospitals may be made to:

KEPRO,   855-408-8557
www.keproqio.com/bene/helpline.aspx

Informal complaints about nursing homes may be raised with:

Long Term Care Ombudsman,   (517) 827-8040 or (866) 485-9393
 Salli Pung, Director   15851 S. US 27, Suite 73
http://mltcop.org/   Lansing. MI 48906

Formal Complaints may be filed with:

Michigan Dept. of Community Health,   Health Facility Complaints
Bureau of Community and Health Systems   P.O. Box 30664
http://www.michigan.gov/lara/0,4601,7-154   Lansing, MI   48909
-63294_63384_70218-339092--,00.html   (800) 882-6006 or
                                                                    (517) 241-0093

Locate an Elder law attorney

National Academy of Elder Law Attorneys   1577 Spring Hill Road, Suite 220,
www.naela.org/MemberDirectory   Vienna, VA   22182.

Locate a Certified Elder law attorney

National Elder Law Foundation   www.nelf.org/findcela.asp

The Area Agencies on Aging are a federally funded resource for aging information and assistance.

Area Agency on Aging Region 1-A   1333 Brewery Park Blvd., Ste. 200
Serves: Detroit, Hamtramck, Highland   Detroit, MI   48207
Park, Grosse Pointes Harper Woods   (313) 446-4444
www.daaa1a.org/DAAA/   Fax: (313) 446-4445

Area Agency on Aging Region 1-B
Serves: Counties of Livingston, Macomb,
Monroe, Oakland, Washtenaw, St. Clair
www.aaa1b.org

29100 Northwestern Hwy., Ste.
400
Southfield, MI   48034
(248) 357-2255   or (800) 852-7795

The Senior Alliance, Region 1-C
Serves: Western and Southern Wayne
County www.aaa1c.org

5454 Venoy Rd,
Wayne, MI 48184
(734) 722-2830 or (800) 815-1112

Social Service agencies offer professional assistance for families in need.

Samaritas - Lutheran Family Services

(313) 823-7700

Catholic Social Services
Wayne County - (855) 882-2736
https://ccsem.org/services-for-seniors

Oakland County - (248) 548-4044
     www.cssoc.org/
Macomb County - (586) 416-2300

Jewish Family Services

(248) 592-2300

**Michigan Association of Homes and
Services for the Aging**
www.mahsahome.org

6512 Centurion Drive, Suite 300
Lansing, MI 48917
(517) 323-3687

The Aging Life Care Association™ –
formerly the National Association of
Professional Geriatric Care Managers
www.caremanager.org

3275 West Ina Road, Suite 130
Tucson, AZ   85741-2198
(520) 881-8008

Further Reading

The Michigan Long Term Care Companion ,
1998, written by Michael Connor and
published by Citizens for Better Care

Available as used book
Amazon.com or Alibris.com

Nursing Homes, Getting Good Care There
164 page book, prepared by The National
Citizens Coalition for Nursing Home
Reform.

Available in Kindle edition on
Amazon.com or as used book on
Amazon or Alibris.com

Moving a Relative with Memory Loss
by Laurie White and Beth Spencer

Available on Amazon.com

Selected Medicare Regulations on Skilled Care

42 *Code of Federal Regulations* (CFR) 409.31 Level of care requirement.

(a) Definition. As used in this section, *skilled nursing* and *skilled rehabilitation services* means services that:

(1) Are ordered by a physician;

(2) Require the skills of technical or professional personnel such as registered nurses, licensed practical (vocational) nurses, physical therapists, occupational therapists, and speech pathologists or audiologists; and

(3) Are furnished directly by, or under the supervision of, such personnel.

(b) Specific conditions for meeting level of care requirements.

(1) The beneficiary must require skilled nursing or skilled rehabilitation services, or both, on a daily basis.

(2) Those services must be furnished for a condition–

(i) For which the beneficiary received inpatient hospital or inpatient CAH services; or

(ii) Which arose while the beneficiary was receiving care in a SNF or swing-bed hospital for a condition for which he or she received inpatient hospital or inpatient CAH services.

(3) The daily skilled services must be ones that, as a practical matter, can only be provided in a SNF, on an inpatient basis.

42 CFR. 409.32 Criteria for skilled services and the need for skilled services.

(a) To be considered a skilled service, the service must be so inherently complex that it can be safely and effectively performed only by, or under the supervision of, professional or technical personnel.

(b) A condition that does not ordinarily require skilled services may require them because of special medical complications. Under those circumstances, a service that is usually nonskilled (such as those listed in § 409.33(d)) may be considered skilled because it must be performed or supervised by skilled nursing or rehabilitation personnel. For example, a plaster cast on a leg does not usually require skilled care. However, if the patient has a preexisting acute skin condition or needs traction, skilled personnel may be needed to adjust traction or watch for complications. In situations of this type, the complications, and the skilled services they require, must be documented by physicians' orders and nursing or therapy notes.

(c) The *restoration potential of a patient is not the deciding factor* in determining whether skilled services are needed. Even if full recovery or medical improvement is not possible, a patient may need skilled services to prevent further deterioration or preserve current capabilities. For example, a terminal cancer patient may need some of the skilled services described in 42 CFR. 409.33.

42 CFR. 409.33 Examples of skilled nursing and rehabilitation services.
(a) Services that could qualify as either skilled nursing or skilled rehabilitation services-
    (1) Overall management and evaluation of care plan.
        (i) When overall management and evaluation of care plan constitute skilled services. The development, management, and evaluation of a patient care plan based on the physician's orders constitute skilled services when, because of the patient's physical or mental condition, those activities require the involvement of technical or professional personnel in order to meet the patient's needs, promote recovery, and ensure medical safety. Those activities include the management of a plan involving a variety of personal care services only when, in light of the patient's condition, the aggregate of those services requires the involvement of technical or professional personnel.
        (ii) Example. An aged patient with a history of diabetes mellitus and angina pectoris who is recovering from an open reduction of a fracture of the neck of the femur requires, among other services, careful skin care, appropriate oral medications, a diabetic diet, an exercise program to preserve muscle tone and body condition, and observation to detect signs of deterioration in his or her condition or complications resulting from restricted, but increasing, mobility. Although any of the required services could be performed by a properly instructed person, such a person would not have the ability to understand the relationship between the services and evaluate the ultimate effect of one service on the other. Since the nature of the patient's condition, age, and immobility create a high potential for serious complications, such an understanding is essential to ensure the patient's recovery and safety. Under these circumstances, the management of the plan of care would require the skills of a nurse even though the individual services are not skilled. Skilled planning and management activities are not always specifically identified in the patient's clinical record. Therefore, if the patient's overall condition supports a finding that recovery and safety can be ensured only if the total care is planned, managed, and evaluated by technical or professional personnel, it is appropriate to infer that skilled services are being provided.
    (2) Observation and assessment of the patient's changing condition-
        (i) When observation and assessment constitute skilled services.

Observation and assessment constitute skilled services when the skills of a technical or professional person are required to identify and evaluate the patient's need for modification of treatment or for additional medical procedures until his or her condition is stabilized.

(ii) Examples. A patient with congestive heart failure may require continuous close observation to detect signs of decompensation, abnormal fluid balance, or adverse effects resulting from prescribed medication(s) that serve as indicators for adjusting therapeutic measures. Similarly, surgical patients transferred from a hospital to an SNF while in the complicated, unstabilized postoperative period, for example, after hip prosthesis or cataract surgery, may need continued close skilled monitoring for postoperative complications and adverse reaction. Patients who, in addition to their physical problems, exhibit acute psychological symptoms such as depression, anxiety, or agitation, may also require skilled observation and assessment by technical or professional personnel to ensure their safety or the safety of others, that is, to observe for indications of suicidal or hostile behavior. The need for services of this type must be documented by physicians' orders or nursing or therapy notes.

(3) Patient education services-

(i) When patient education services constitute skilled services. Patient education services are skilled services if the use of technical or professional personnel is necessary to teach a patient self-maintenance.

(ii) Examples. A patient who has had a recent leg amputation needs skilled rehabilitation services provided by technical or professional personnel to provide gait training and to teach prosthesis care. Similarly, a patient newly diagnosed with diabetes requires instruction from technical or professional personnel to learn the self-administration of insulin or foot-care precautions.

(b) Services that qualify as skilled nursing services.

(1) Intravenous or intramuscular injections and intravenous feeding.

(2) Enteral feeding that comprises at least 26 per cent of daily calorie requirements and provides at least 501 milliliters of fluid per day.

(3) Nasopharyngeal and tracheostomy aspiration;

(4) Insertion and sterile irrigation and replacement of suprapubic catheters;

(5) Application of dressings involving prescription medications and aseptic techniques;

(6) Treatment of extensive decubitus ulcers or other widespread skin disorder;

(7) Heat treatments which have been specifically ordered by a physician as part of active treatment and which require observation by nurses to adequately evaluate

the patient's progress;

(8) Initial phases of a regimen involving administration of medical gases;

(9) Rehabilitation nursing procedures, including the related teaching and adaptive aspects of nursing, that are part of active treatment, e.g., the institution and supervision of bowel and bladder training programs.

(c) Services which would qualify as skilled rehabilitation services.

(1) Ongoing assessment of rehabilitation needs and potential: Services concurrent with the management of a patient care plan, including tests and measurements of range of motion, strength, balance, coordination, endurance, functional ability, activities of daily living, perceptual deficits, speech and language or hearing disorders;

(2) Therapeutic exercises or activities: Therapeutic exercises or activities which, because of the type of exercises employed or the condition of the patient, must be performed by or under the supervision of a qualified physical therapist or occupational therapist to ensure the safety of the patient and the effectiveness of the treatment;

(3) Gait evaluation and training: Gait evaluation and training furnished to restore function in a patient whose ability to walk has been impaired by neurological, muscular, or skeletal abnormality;

(4) Range of motion exercises: Range of motion exercises which are part of the active treatment of a specific disease state which has resulted in a loss of, or restriction of, mobility (as evidenced by a therapist's notes showing the degree of motion lost and the degree to be restored);

(5) Maintenance therapy; Maintenance therapy, when the specialized knowledge and judgment of a qualified therapist is required to design and establish a maintenance program based on an initial evaluation and periodic reassessment of the patient's needs, and consistent with the patient's capacity and tolerance. For example, a patient with Parkinson's disease who has not been under a rehabilitation regimen may require the services of a qualified therapist to determine what type of exercises will contribute the most to the maintenance of his present level of functioning.

(6) Ultrasound, short-wave, and microwave therapy treatment by a qualified physical therapist;

(7) Hot pack, hydrocollator, infrared treatments, paraffin baths, and whirlpool; Hot pack hydrocollator, infrared treatments, paraffin baths, and whirlpool in particular cases where the patient's condition is complicated by circulatory deficiency, areas of desensitization, open wounds, fractures, or other complications, and the skills, knowledge, and judgment of a qualified physical therapist are required; and

(8) Services of a speech pathologist or audiologist when necessary for the

restoration of function in speech or hearing.

(d) Personal care services. Personal care services which do <u>not</u> require the skills of qualified technical or professional personnel are not skilled services except under the circumstances specified in § 409.32(b). Personal care services include, but are not limited to, the following:

(1) Administration of routine oral medications, eye drops, and ointments;

(2) General maintenance care of colostomy and ileostomy;

(3) Routine services to maintain satisfactory functioning of indwelling bladder catheters;

(4) Changes of dressings for noninfected postoperative or chronic conditions;

(5) Prophylactic and palliative skin care, including bathing and application of creams, or treatment of minor skin problems;

(6) Routine care of the incontinent patient, including use of diapers and protective sheets;

(7) General maintenance care in connection with a plaster cast;

(8) Routine care in connection with braces and similar devices;

(9) Use of heat as a palliative and comfort measure, such as whirlpool and hydrocollator;

(10) Routine administration of medical gases after a regimen of therapy has been established;

(11) Assistance in dressing, eating, and going to the toilet;

(12) Periodic turning and positioning in bed; and

(13) General supervision of exercises which have been taught to the patient; including the actual carrying out of maintenance programs, i.e., the performance of the repetitive exercises required to maintain function do not require the skills of a therapist and would not constitute skilled rehabilitation services (see paragraph (c) of this section). Similarly, repetitious exercises to improve gait, maintain strength, or endurance; passive exercises to maintain range of motion in paralyzed extremities, which are not related to a specific loss of function; and assistive walking do not constitute skilled rehabilitation services.

The Seven Doors To Medicaid

Does a person need a nursing home? You can use the same test or "screen" that the Michigan Medicaid department does: The Seven Doors To Medicaid.

This screen will help you determine whether your patient or family member has a nursing home level of care need.

Of course, finding that a persons's "level of care need" is sufficient for Medicaid to pay for a person's care in a nursing home, does not mean there are no alternatives to the nursing home. Many times there are. However, Medicaid will only pay a nursing home. It will not pay the cost of an alternative such as an assisted living facility.

One further note here. While the "Medicaid MiChoice Waiver" program will pay for care in alternative settings, it is a different program. It does not pay the complete facility cost. It has a waiting list. It does not use the 7 Doors Screen. The program requires an assessment of the person's needs and there is a waiting list.

The Seven Doors to Medicaid screen follows on the next pages.

Seven Doors To Medicaid

Michigan Department of Community Health

Michigan Medicaid Nursing Facility Level of Care Determination

Applicant's Name: Field 1 _____ (First) _____ (M.I.) _____
(Last)

Medicaid ID: Field 2

Date of Birth: Field 3 / _____ / _____
00 / 00 / 0000

Provider Type: Field 4 **Medicaid ID:** Field 5

Provider Contact Name: Field 6 _____ (First) _____
(Last)

Provider Day Phone: (Field 7) _____ - _____

Door 1: Activities of Daily Living

A. Bed Mobility: How the applicant moves to and from lying position, turns side to side, and positions body while in bed (sleeping surface).

Field 8 ☐ **Independent**
No help or oversight, OR help or oversight provided only 1 or 2 times during last 7 days.

Field 9 ☐ **Supervision**
Oversight, encouragement or cueing provided 3 or more times during last 7 days, OR supervision 3 or more times plus physical assistance provided only 1 or 2 times during last 7 days.

Field 10 ☐ **Limited Assistance**
Applicant highly involved in activity, received physical help in guided maneuvering of limbs or other non-weight-bearing assistance 3 or more times, OR more help provided only 1 or 2 times during last 7 days.

Field 11 ☐ **Extensive Assistance**
While the applicant performed part of activity over last 7-day period, help of following types(s) provided 3 or more times:
- Weight-bearing support
- Full performance by another during part, but not all, of last 7 days

Field 12 ☐ **Total Dependence**
Full performance of activity by another during entire 7 days.

Field 13 ☐ **Activity did not occur** during entire 7 days (regardless of ability).

B. Transfers: How the applicant moves between surfaces, to/from bed (sleeping surface), chair, wheelchair, standing position (exclude to/from bath/toilet).

Field 14 ☐ **Independent**
No help or oversight, OR help or oversight provided only 1 or 2 times during last 7 days.

Field 15 ☐ **Supervision**
Oversight, encouragement or cueing provided 3 or more times during last 7 days, OR supervision 3 or more times plus physical assistance provided only 1 or 2 times during last 7 days.

Field 16 ☐ **Limited Assistance**
Applicant highly involved in activity, received physical help in guided maneuvering of limbs or other non-weight-bearing assistance 3 or more times, OR more help provided only 1 or 2 times during last 7 days.

Field 17 ☐ **Extensive Assistance**
While the applicant performed part of activity over last 7-day period, help of following types(s) provided 3 or more times:
  • Weight-bearing support
  • Full performance by another during part, but not all, of last 7 days

Field 18 ☐ **Total Dependence**
Full performance of activity by another during entire 7 days.

Field 19 ☐ **Activity did not occur** during entire 7 days (regardless of ability).

    C. Toilet Use: How the applicant uses the toilet room (or commode, bedpan, urinal), transfers on/off toilet, cleanses, changes pad, manages ostomy or catheter, and adjusts clothes.

Field 20 ☐ **Independent**
No help or oversight, OR help or oversight provided only 1 or 2 times during last 7 days.

Field 21 ☐ **Supervision**
Oversight, encouragement or cueing provided 3 or more times during last 7 days, OR supervision 3 or more times plus physical assistance provided only 1 or 2 times during last 7 days.

Field 22 ☐ **Limited Assistance**
Applicant highly involved in activity, received physical help in guided maneuvering of limbs or other non-weight-bearing assistance 3 or more times, OR more help provided only 1 or 2 times during last 7 days.

Field 23 ☐ **Extensive Assistance**
While the applicant performed part of activity over last 7-day period, help of following types(s) provided 3 or more times:
  • Weight-bearing support
  • Full performance by another during part, but not all, of last 7 days

Field 24 ☐ **Total Dependence**
Full performance of activity by another during entire 7 days.

Field 25 ☐ **Activity did not occur** during entire 7 days (regardless of ability).

    D. Eating: How the applicant eats and drinks (regardless of skill). Includes intake of nourishment by other means (i.e., tube feeding, total parenteral nutrition).

Field 26 ☐ **Independent**
No help or oversight, OR help or oversight provided only 1 or 2 times during last 7 days.

Field 27 ☐ **Supervision**
Oversight, encouragement or cueing provided 3 or more times during last 7 days, OR supervision 3 or more times plus physical assistance provided only 1 or 2 times during last 7 days.

Field 28 ☐ **Limited Assistance**
Applicant received physical help in guided maneuvering of limbs or other assistance 3 or more times, OR more help provided only 1 or 2 times during last 7 days.

Field 29 ☐ **Extensive Assistance**
While the applicant performed part of activity over last 7-day period, help of the following type provided 3 or more times:
- Full performance by another during part, but not all, of last 7 days

Field 30 ☐ **Total Dependence**
Full performance of activity by another during entire 7 days.

Field 31 ☐ **Activity did not occur** during entire 7 days (regardless of ability).

Scoring Door 1: The applicant must score at least six points to qualify under Door 1.

(A) Bed Mobility, (B) Transfers, and (C) Toilet Use:
- Independent or Supervision = 1
- Limited Assistance = 3
- Extensive Assistance or Total Dependence = 4
- Activity Did Not Occur = 8

(D) Eating:
- Independent or Supervision = 1
- Limited Assistance = 2
- Extensive Assistance or Total Dependence = 3
- Activity Did Not Occur = 8

Door 2: Cognitive Performance (Does the applicant have any problems with memory or making decisions?)

A. Short-term memory okay (seems/appears to recall after 5 minutes)

Field 32 ☐ **Memory Okay**

Field 33 ☐ **Memory Problem**

B. Cognitive skills for daily decision-making (made decisions regarding tasks of daily life for last 7 days).

Field 34 ☐ **Independent**
The applicant's decisions were consistent and reasonable (reflecting lifestyle, culture, values); the applicant organized daily routine and made decisions in a consistent, reasonable, and organized fashion.

Field 35 ☐ **Modified Independent**
The applicant organized daily routine and made safe decisions in familiar situations, but experienced some difficulty in decision-making when faced with new tasks or situations.

Field 36 ☐ **Moderately Impaired**
The applicant's decisions were poor; the applicant required reminders, cues, and supervision in planning, organizing, and correcting daily routines.

Field 37 ☐ **Severely Impaired**
The applicant's decision-making was severely impaired, the applicant never (or rarely) made decisions.

C. Making self understood (expressing information content, however able).

Field 38 ☐ **Understood**
The applicant expresses ideas clearly, without difficulty.

Field 39 ☐ **Usually Understood**
The applicant has difficulty finding the right words or finishing thoughts, resulting in delayed responses. If given time, little or no prompting required.

Field 40 ☐ **Sometimes Understood**
The applicant has limited ability, but is able to express concrete requests regarding at least basic needs (i.e., food, drink, sleep, toilet).

Field 41 ☐ **Rarely/Never Understood**
At best, understanding is limited to interpretation of highly individual, applicant-specific sounds or body language (i.e., indicated presence of pain or need to toilet).

Scoring Door 2: The applicant must score under one of the following three options to qualify under Door 2.

1. "Severely Impaired" in Decision Making.

2. "Yes" for Memory Problem, and Decision Making is "Moderately Impaired" or "Severely Impaired."

3. "Yes" for Memory Problem, and Making Self Understood is "Sometimes Understood" or "Rarely/Never Understood."

Door 3: Physician Involvement (Is the applicant under the care of a physician for treatment of an unstable medical condition?)

Field 42 **A.** **Physician Visits:** In the last 14 days, how many days has the physician, or authorized assistant or practitioner, examined the applicant? **Do not** count emergency room exams. Enter "0" if none.

☐☐

Field 43 **B.** **Physician Orders:** In the last 14 days, how many days has the physician, or authorized assistant or practitioner, changed the applicant's orders? **Do not** include drug or treatment order renewals without change. Enter "0" if none.

☐☐

> **Scoring Door 3:** The applicant must meet either of the following to qualify under Door 3.
>
> 1. At least one Physician Visit exam AND at least four Physician Order changes in the last 14 days, OR
>
> 2. At least two Physician Visit exams AND at least two Physician Order changes in the last 14 days.

Door 4: Treatments and Conditions (Has the applicant in the last 14 days received any of the following health treatments, or demonstrated any of the following health conditions?) <u>Complete each item below, either Yes or No</u>.

		Yes	No
Field 44/45	A. Stage 3-4 pressure sores	☐	☐
Field 46/47	B. Intravenous or parenteral feedings	☐	☐
Field 48/49	C. Intravenous medications	☐	☐
Field 50/51	D. End-stage care	☐	☐
Field 52/53	E. Daily tracheostomy care, daily respiratory care, daily suctioning	☐	☐
Field 54/55	F. Pneumonia within the last 14 days	☐	☐
Field 56/57	G. Daily oxygen therapy	☐	☐
Field 58/59	H. Daily insulin with two order changes in last 14 days	☐	☐
Field 60/61	I. Peritoneal or hemodialysis	☐	☐

> **Scoring Door 4:** The applicant must score "yes" in at least one of the nine categories and have a continuing need to qualify under Door 4.

Door 5:   Skilled Rehabilitation Therapies (Is the applicant currently receiving any skilled rehabilitation therapies?)

Record the total minutes each of the following therapies was administered or scheduled (for at least 15 minutes a day) in the last 7 days. Enter "0" if none or less than 15 minutes daily.
        A = Total number of minutes provided in last 7 days
        B = Total number of minutes scheduled but not yet administered

		A	B
1.	Speech Therapy		
	Fields	62	63
2.	Occupational Therapy		
	Fields	64	65
3.	Physical Therapy		
	Fields	66	67

Example:

A	B
2 1 0	6 0

Scoring Door 5: The applicant must have required at least 45 minutes of active ST, OT or PT (scheduled or delivered) in the last 7 days and continues to require skilled rehabilitation therapies to qualify under Door 5.

Door 6: Behavior (Has the applicant displayed any challenging behaviors in the last 7 days?)

Behavioral Code:
- 0 = Behavior not exhibited in last 7 days
- 1 = Behavior of this type occurred 1 to 3 days in last 7 days
- 2 = Behavior of this type occurred 4 to 6 days, but less than daily
- 3 = Behavior of this type occurred daily

Behavioral Symptoms:

		0	1	2	3
A.	**Wandering** - Moved with no rational purpose, seemingly oblivious to needs and safety.				
	Fields	68	69	70	71
B.	**Verbally Abusive** - Others were threatened, screamed at, cursed at.				
	Fields	72	73	74	75
C.	**Physically Abusive** - Others were hit, shoved, scratched, sexually abused.				
	Fields	76	77	78	79
D.	**Socially Inappropriate/Disruptive** - Made disruptive sounds, noisiness, screaming, self-abusive acts, inappropriate sexual behavior or disrobing in public, smeared or threw food/feces, hoarded or rummaged through others' belongings.				
	Fields	80	81	82	83
E.	**Resists Care** - Resisted taking medications or injections, ADL assistance or eating.				
	Fields	84	85	86	87

Problem Condition Code: If present at any point in last 7 days, code either Yes or No.

Problem Conditions:

	Yes	No
A. Delusions	☐	☐
Fields	88	89
B. Hallucinations	☐	☐
Fields	90	91

Scoring Door 6: The applicant must score under one of the following 2 options to qualify under Door 6.

1. A "Yes" for either delusions or hallucinations within the last 7 days.

2. The applicant must have exhibited any one of the following behaviors for at least 4 of the last 7 days (including daily): Wandering, Verbally Abusive, Physically Abusive, Socially Inappropriate/Disruptive, or Resisted Care.

Door 7:   Service Dependency

The applicant is currently being served by either the MI Choice Program, PACE program or Medicaid reimbursed nursing facility.

Field 92   ☐   **Program participant for at least one year** and requires ongoing services to maintain current functional status. You may combine time the applicant received services across the three programs. No other community, residential or informal services are available to meet the applicant's needs.

Field 93   ☐   **Not a program participant for one year.**

Scoring Door 7: The applicant must be a current participant and demonstrate service dependency to qualify under Door 7.

---

www.ingramcontent.com/pod-product-compliance
Lightning Source LLC
Chambersburg PA
CBHW081657270326
41933CB00017B/3196